Aids to Postgraduate Medicine

J. L. Burton MD BSc FRCP
Professor of Dermatology, Bristol Royal Infirmary, Bristol

C. J. Healey MB ChB MRCP
Research Registrar, John Radcliffe Hospital, Oxford

SIXTH EDITION

CHURCHILL LIVINGSTONE
EDINBURGH LONDON MADRID MELBOURNE NEW YORK AND TOKYO 1994

CHURCHILL LIVINGSTONE
Medical Division of Longman Group UK Limited

Distributed in the United States of America by
Churchill Livingstone Inc., 650 Avenue of the
Americas, New York, N.Y. 10011, and by
associated companies, branches and
representatives throughout the world.

First edition 1970
Second edition 1974
Third edition 1978
Fourth edition 1983
Fifth edition 1988
Sixth edition 1994
   Reprinted 1995

ISBN 0 443 04913 0

British Library Cataloguing in Publication Data
A catalogue record for this book is available
from the British Library.

Library of Congress Cataloguing in Publication
Data
A catalog record for this book is available from
the Library of Congress.

The
publisher's
policy is to use
**paper manufactured
from sustainable forests**

Produced by Longman Singapore Publishers (Pte) Ltd.
Printed in Singapore

Preface

This book is intended primarily to provide a compact aid to revision for candidates taking postgraduate examinations in general medicine. We hope it will also prove useful to other doctors wishing to refresh their memories of the diagnostic possibilities in a particular case. It should also be helpful in the preparation of case-presentations.

This edition has been completely revised. Many of the lists have been updated, a few which had become obsolete have been omitted, and many new topics have been included, ranging from amnesia to molecular biology.

Many people have given helpful advice and suggestions and we are grateful for their help.

Bristol   J.L.B.
Oxford   C.J.H.
1994

Contents

Preface vii

1. Cardiology 1
2. Chest disease 22
3. Gastroenterology 43
4. Haematology 72
5. Neurology 100
6. Endocrine and bone disease 136
7. Renal disease 165
8. Rheumatology 181
9. Dermatology 196
10. Venereology 215
11. Immunology 218
12. Genetics and molecular biology 225
13. Pyrexia and hypothermia 235
14. Clinical chemistry 237
15. Statistics 242

Bibliography 247

Index 253

Cardiology

ARTERIAL PULSE

Causes of tachycardia
1. Sinus tachycardia (q.v.)
2. Supraventricular (atrial or nodal) tachycardia
3. Atrial flutter
4. Atrial fibrillation
5. Ventricular tachycardia
6. Ventricular flutter

Causes of sinus tachycardia
1. Hyperdynamic circulation (q.v.)
2. Congestive cardiac failure
3. Constrictive pericarditis
4. Drugs (adrenaline, atropine, nitrites, etc.)
5. Hypovolaemic shock (acute haemorrhage, etc.)

Causes of hyperdynamic circulation
1. Exercise or emotion (anxiety, fright, etc.)
2. Pregnancy
3. Anaemia
4. Pyrexia
5. Thyrotoxicosis
6. AV aneurysm
7. Paget's disease
8. Beri-beri
9. Hepatic failure
10. Hypercapnia
11. Erythroderma
12. Vasodilator drugs

Causes of a slow regular pulse
1. Sinus bradycardia (q.v.)
2. Complete heart block
3. 2 : 1 AV block
4. Atrial flutter or fibrillation with high degree of AV block
5. Sinus arrest with idionodal rhythm

Causes of sinus bradycardia
1. Congenital
2. Physical training
3. Convalescence from fever
4. Soon after myocardial infarction
5. Sinoatrial disorder ('sick sinus syndrome')
6. Jaundice
7. Myxoedema
8. Hypothermia
9. Raised intracranial pressure
10. Drugs (digitalis, betablockers, hypotensives)
11. Rapid rise in blood pressure
12. Transiently increased vagal tone (e.g. vomiting)

Causes of a 'dropped beat'
1. Sinoatrial block
2. Blocked atrial extrasystole
3. 2nd degree heart block

Causes of an irregular pulse
1. Extrasystole (ventricular or supraventricular)
2. Atrial fibrillation
3. Sinus arrhythmia
4. Atrial flutter with varying block
5. 2nd degree heart block

Irregularity of volume also occurs in pulsus paradoxus and pulsus alternans

Causes of atrial fibrillation
1. Rheumatic heart disease, especially MS
2. Thyrotoxicosis
3. Myocardial ischaemia
4. Hypertension
5. Idiopathic ('lone') fibrillation, sick sinus syndrome or mitral valve prolapse
6. Chronic constrictive pericarditis
7. Atrial septal defect (over age 50)
8. Heart muscle disease (esp. alcoholic)
9. Wolff–Parkinson–White syndrome
10. Rarely atrial myxoma, bacterial endocarditis, acute pericarditis, Ca bronchus, cor pulmonale, post-pneumonectomy, head injury

Sick sinus syndrome
There is considerable overlap between the physiological bradycardia seen in athletes, and that occurring in patients with the sick sinus syndrome, and profound bradycardia and even sinus arrest can occur in normal young people.

Definition of established sinoatrial disorder
A chronic sinus rate below 50 with one or more of the following:
1. Sinus pause of 2 seconds or more
2. Atrial rate below 40 (usually with junctional rhythm)
3. Paroxysmal tachycardia (AF, atrial flutter, or atrial or ventricular tachycardia)

Potential sinoatrial disorder
A chronic unexplained sinus bradycardia in the absence of the above factors

HEART BLOCK

Classification
1. Sinoatrial block
2. AV block
   1st degree, PR > 0.2 sec
   2nd degree
   (i) Dropped beats
       Fixed PR
       Varying PR (Wenkebach)
   (ii) Fixed AV relationship (2 : 1, 3 : 1, etc.)
   3rd degree, Complete
3. Bundle branch block
4. Intraventricular block

Causes
1. Congenital (usually AV nodal)
2. Idiopathic
3. Ischaemic heart disease
4. Aortic stenosis
5. Drugs (digitalis) or iatrogenic ablation
6. Cardiomyopathy (including myocardial infiltration and collagen-vascular disease)
7. Myocarditis (rheumatic, diphtheritic)
8. Rarely trauma, tumour, syphilis, hypertension

VENTRICULAR PRE-EXCITATION

Wolff–Parkinson–White syndrome is due to congenital accessory pathway for AV conduction with premature ventricular activation
    ECG shows short PR, wide QRS and slurred delta wave at onset of QRS

Arrhythmias caused by WPW syndrome
1. Paroxysmal tachycardia
2. Paroxysmal atrial fibrillation
3. Sinus node dysfunction

Digitalis should not be given for AF in this condition, as it may provoke VF

The *Lown–Ganong–Levine syndrome* is a 'forme fruste' of WPW, with a short PR, but normal QRS and no delta wave

Idiopathic long QT syndrome is due to neural degeneration of the conduction system. It is characterized by long QT, recurrent syncope, ventricular arrhythmias and sudden death. It may result from electrolyte imbalance, neurological disease and toxicity from cardiac or psychotropic drugs

JUGULAR VENOUS PULSE (JVP)

Normal jugular venous pulse wave

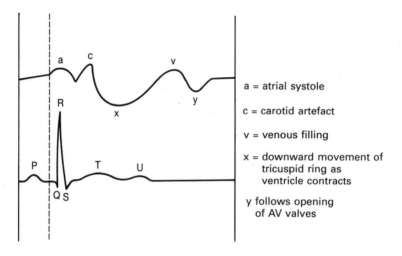

a = atrial systole

c = carotid artefact

v = venous filling

x = downward movement of tricuspid ring as ventricle contracts

y follows opening of AV valves

Abnormalities of venous pulse wave
1. *Giant 'a' waves*
    (i)   pulmonary hypertension
    (ii) severe pulmonary stenosis
    (iii) tricuspid stenosis
2. *Cannon waves*
    (i)   Regular: Nodal rhythm
    (ii) Irregular: Complete heart block
                    Multiple extrasystoles
3. *Absent 'a' waves:* atrial fibrillation
4. *Independent 'a' waves:* complete heart block
5. *Large 'v' waves:* tricuspid incompetence (confirm by palpation of systolic impulse in liver)

6. *Deep 'y' descent:* any cause of very high JVP especially constrictive pericarditis
7. *Slow 'y' descent:* tricuspid stenosis

CAUSES OF ELEVATED JVP

1. Hyperdynamic circulation (p. 1)
2. R ventricular failure
3. Obstruction of superior vena cava (non-pulsatile)
4. Tricuspid stenosis or incompetence
5. Pericardial effusion or constrictive pericarditis
6. Fluid overload (esp. i.v. infusion)
7. Very slow heart rate

AUSCULTATION

HEART SOUNDS

1. Valve closure
1st heart sound (mitral and tricuspid valves)
      (i) Loud in: Mitral stenosis
                        Hyperdynamic circulation
                        Tachycardia
     (ii) Normally split in tricuspid area on inspiration
2nd heart sound (aortic and pulmonary valves)
      (i) Normally split on inspiration, especially in children
     (ii) Loud narrowly split P_2 in pulmonary hypertension
    (iii) Soft widely split P_2 in pulmonary stenosis
    (iv) Widely split in RBBB
     (v) Widely split fixed P_2 in ASD
    (vi) Paradoxically split P_2 (narrows on inspiration) in LBBB and rarely in aortic stenosis and severe hypertension

2. Opening snap
Heard only with AV valve stenosis
Indicates mobile AV valve
Mitral opening snap in mitral stenosis is maximal medial to apex, louder during expiration, thereby differentiated from split P_2
Closeness to 2nd sound indicates severity of stenosis

3. Ejection sounds
Early systolic clicks due to aortic or pulmonary stenosis, or to dilatation of pulmonary artery or aorta in pulmonary or systemic hypertension
Mid- or late-systolic clicks due to mitral valve prolapse

4. Ventricular filling sounds (Triple rhythm)

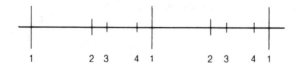

Diastolic sounds are due to:
   (i) 3rd heart sound (rapid ventricular filling)
  (ii) atrial (4th) sound (forceful atrial contraction)
 (iii) summation of both
3rd heart sound is normal in young people. Occurs in older people in:
   (i) R or L ventricular failure
  (ii) Mitral or tricuspid regurgitation
 (iii) Constrictive pericarditis (early and sharp)
Atrial sound is abnormal, occurs in resistance to LV filling, e.g. hypertensive LVH, aortic stenosis
Summation sound is normal during tachycardia

5. Extracardiac sounds
Usually pericardial in origin, vary with respiration and posture

HEART MURMURS

High-pitched indicate large pressure difference across small orifice, e.g. AS
Low-pitched indicate small pressure difference across large orifice, e.g. MI

1. Systolic
   (i) *Midsystolic ejection murmurs*
      Aortic
         a. Aortic stenosis—confirmed by narrow pulse pressure and thrill (patient leaning forward in expiration)
         b. Increased flow rate
         c. Valve thickening or sclerosis without stenosis
         d. Post-valvar dilatation, e.g. hypertension or aortic aneurysm
      Pulmonary
         a. Functional, especially in young people
         b. Pulmonary stenosis
         c. Increased flow rate ASD, TAPVD (total anomalous pulmonary venous drainage), hyperdynamic circulation
         d. Post-valvar dilatation, e.g. pulmonary hypertension

(ii) *Pansystolic murmurs*
Extend from 1st to 2nd sound
    a. Mitral regurgitation—propagated into axilla (In mitral valve prolapse there may be a late systolic murmur)
    b. Tricuspid regurgitation—increases with inspiration, soft unless pulmonary hypertension is present
    c. VSD—3rd or 4th LICS. Thrill in 90%

Causes of a loud systolic murmur with a thrill
  (i) At apex—mitral regurgitation
  (ii) At 4th LICS—VSD
  (iii) At pulmonary area—pulmonary stenosis
  (iv) At aortic area—aortic stenosis

2. **Diastolic**
  (i) *Mitral or tricuspid stenosis*
    Mitral stenosis—use bell, lightly applied at apex, with patient on L side in expiration
    Tricuspid stenosis—murmur louder on inspiration
  (ii) *Mitral or tricuspid thickening*, e.g. Carey–Coombs murmur of active rheumatic carditis
  (iii) *Increased AV flow rate*
    Mitral in VSD and PDA (patent ductus arteriosus)
    Tricuspid in ASD and TAPVD
  (iv) *Aortic or pulmonary regurgitation*
    Aortic regurgitation—often missed. Listen with diaphragm all down L sternal edge for soft 'whispered R' murmur with patient leaning forward in expiration
    Pulmonary regurgitation—usually due to pulmonary hypertension
    Austin–**Fl**nt murmur (functional mitral stenosis) may occur in **A**ortic **I**ncompetence
    Graha**M**–**S**teell murmur (pulmonary regurgitation) may occur in **M**itral **S**tenosis with pulmonary hypertension

3. **Continuous** ('Machinery murmur')
  (i) Patent ductus arteriosus (2nd LICS or under clavicle)
  (ii) Aorticopulmonary septal defect (2nd or 3rd LICS)
  (iii) Pulmonary AV fistula (over lung fields)
  (iv) Bronchial artery anastomosis in pulmonary atresia
  (v) Artificial ductus (Blalock or Waterston shunt)
  (vi) Venous hum
  (vii) Prosthetic valve

Effect of respiration on murmurs
Inspiration increases stroke volume of R ventricle, therefore increases intensity of TS, TI and PS

Inspiration increases vascular volume of lungs and decreases stroke volume of L ventricle, therefore decreases intensity of MS, MI, AS and AI

Effect of posture on murmurs and cardiac sounds
Mitral systolic and diastolic murmurs. Accentuated in L lateral position
Aortic murmurs, ejection clicks and pericardial rub. Accentuated when sitting up
Functional systolic murmurs. Accentuated when lying down
Venous hum (in supraclavicular space). Heard only when upright
Accentuated by turning head away from side being examined

Effect of drugs on murmurs
Drugs increasing arteriolar resistance will decrease systolic ejection murmurs and increase regurgitant murmurs at all valves
Vasodilators have the opposite effect

Characteristics of innocent systolic murmurs in childhood
1. No other abnormality detected
2. No thrill
3. Usually short, of low frequency, and in early or midsystole
4. Not localized to a specific area, and not radiating outside praecordium
5. Intensity often varies with change in posture

RHEUMATIC FEVER

Revised Jones criteria for diagnosis—two major or one major and two minor

Major
1. Carditis
2. Polyarthritis
3. Erythema marginatum
4. Subcutaneous nodules
5. Chorea

Minor
1. Fever
2. Arthalgia
3. Past history of rheumatic fever
4. Raised acute phase reactants
5. ECG, prolonged PR interval

Other
Evidence of streptococcal infection (absence makes diagnosis doubtful)

MITRAL STENOSIS

The signs vary with the severity of the stenosis and the increase in pulmonary hypertension

1. The *loud first heart sound* is due to the closing snap of the mitral valve
2. The *opening snap* follows the second heart sound. It is high-pitched, widely transmitted, best heard to the left of the sternum near the base of the heart
3. The *diastolic murmur* is long and rumbling, with presystolic accentuation due to atrial systole. The longer the murmur, the more severe the stenosis, but with pulmonary hypertension the murmur becomes shorter

Presystolic accentuation is often a sign of pure stenosis, but is absent in atrial fibrillation

In MS with pulmonary hypertension:

1. The patient is usually thin, with peripheral cyanosis, cool extremities and low volume pulse. A mitral facies indicates a low cardiac output
2. JVP is raised with a prominent 'a' wave (in sinus rhythm)
3. There may be cardiac enlargement with a R ventricular heave
4. The auscultatory signs of MS become less obvious
5. Calcification of the valve may eliminate the opening snap, but should not affect the murmur
6. Low cardiac output may eliminate the murmur, but should not affect the opening snap

In MS with atrial fibrillation:

Establish the time of onset, and the patient's tolerance of the AF

1. If the onset was not noticed by the patient, this indicates either mild MS or the presence of pulmonary hypertension
2. The earlier the AF occurs, the worse the prognosis. If AF has not occurred by age 50 the MS is probably mild

In mixed MS and MI:

1. If there is more stenosis than incompetence, there is less systolic back-flow, and less diastolic forward-flow
2. If there is more incompetence than stenosis, there is more systolic back-flow and more systolic forward-flow
3. Because of this compensatory effect, the symptoms tend to remain constant, but the signs vary with the severity of the incompetence
4. A loud systolic murmur may be heard in mild MI, but presystolic accentuation of the diastolic murmur excludes significant MI

MITRAL INCOMPETENCE

Causes
1. Rheumatic fever (probably about 20% of cases in UK)
2. Mitral valve prolapse
3. Degenerative valve changes, e.g. tear, myxomatous degeneration or associated with connective-tissue disease (Marfan's, osteogenesis imperfecta, Ehlers–Danlos)
4. Infective endocarditis (may be a cause or a complication)
5. Ischaemia, especially posterior infarct, with papillary muscle damage
6. Congenital
7. Calcification of the mitral ring (rare, occurs in elderly women)
8. Trauma (e.g. severe blow to the chest)

The 'click-murmur' syndrome
Haemodynamically insignificant mitral incompetence

Causes
As for MI (see above), but mitral valve prolapse is the commonest
On echocardiography, 15% of apparently normal young women have this condition

Clinical features
Symptoms: None, or cardiac neurosis (iatrogenic)
Signs: Late systolic mitral murmur of a 'honking' quality, with or without a late systolic click
ECG: May be normal, or show P mitrale, or ST and T wave changes suggestive of ischaemia

Complications
1. Infective endocarditis
2. Acute disruption of the mitral valve (spontaneous or traumatic)
3. Coronary artery disease (possibly due to minor dysfunction of the papillary muscle)
4. Ventricular arrhythmia
5. Transient cerebral ischaemia

AORTIC REGURGITATION

Causes
Cusp: Distortion
              Rheumatic
              Rheumatoid
           Perforation
              Infective endocarditis
              Trauma

Ring: Dilation
          Dissecting aneurysm or hypertension
          Marfan's syndrome
          Syphilis
          Ankylosing spondylitis
Others: Failure of prosthetic valve
          VSD
          Ruptured sinus of Valsalva

Differential diagnosis of valvular disease
1. Functional murmur
2. Atrial myxoma
3. Hypertrophic cardiomyopathy
4. Ruptured papillary muscle or chordae tendineae
5. Aneurysm of sinus of Valsalva

HEART FAILURE

Definition: A state in which the heart fails to meet the metabolic and oxygen needs of the body under varying conditions, assuming the venous return is adequate

VALSALVA MANOEUVRE

Normal response of pulse and BP

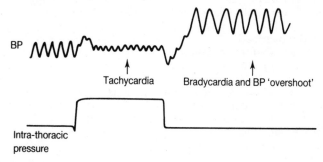

BP

↑
Tachycardia

↑
Bradycardia and BP 'overshoot'

Intra-thoracic
pressure

Cardiac failure causes a square wave response

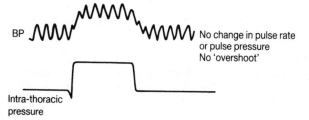

BP

No change in pulse rate
or pulse pressure
No 'overshoot'

Intra-thoracic
pressure

CAUSES OF LV FAILURE

1. **Pressure overload**
    (i)   Hypertension
    (ii) Aortic stenosis
    (iii) Coarctation

2. **Volume overload**
    (i)   Aortic or mitral regurgitation
    (ii) VSD or PDA
    (iii) AV fistula or anaemia

3. **Myocardial ischaemia**
    (i)   Coronary artery disease
    (ii) Severe anaemia
    (iii) Tachycardia

4. **Primary myocardial disease**
    (i)   Myocarditis
    (ii) Cardiomyopathy

CAUSES OF RV FAILURE

1. **Pressure overload**
    (i)   Pulmonary hypertension secondary to LVF or MS
    (ii) Cor pulmonale
    (iii) Severe pulmonary stenosis

2. **Volume overload**
    (i)   Tricuspid regurgitation
    (ii) ASD or TAPVD

Causes of generalized cardiomegaly on chest X-ray
    1. Congestive cardiac failure
    2. Multiple valve lesions
    3. Pericardial effusion
    4. Cardiomyopathy
    5. Myocarditis
    6. Ebstein's disease
    7. Hyperdynamic circulation
    8. Complete heart block

CARDIOMYOPATHY

Definition: Heart muscle disease of unknown cause. If the underlying disease is identified, it becomes 'specific heart muscle disease', even if the aetiology of the underlying disease (e.g. amyloidosis) is obscure. These terms have replaced the former classification of primary and secondary cardiomyopathy. Myocardial disease secondary to structural changes (e.g. valvular lesions) or hypertension is excluded

CAUSES OF CARDIOMYOPATHY

1. *Dilated cardiomyopathy* (formerly called 'congestive'). Isolated cardiomegaly, gallop rhythm and idiopathic heart failure
2. *Hypertrophic cardiomyopathy* (HOCM) (formerly called 'obstructive')

These two types account for 98% of primary cases in UK

3. *Restrictive cardiomyopathy*
   Endomyocardial fibrosis. May progress to the obliterative form

SPECIFIC HEART MUSCLE DISEASE

Most of these fall into the same functional class as dilated cardiomyopathy, unless there is severe infiltration, as in amyloid or glycogen storage disease

1. *Infective*
   - (i) Viral (post-myocarditis)
   - (ii) Bacterial, e.g. diphtheria toxin
   - (iii) Protozoal, e.g. schistosomiasis
     toxoplasmosis
     trypanosomiasis (Chagas')
2. *Metabolic and endocrine*
   - (i) Pregnancy and puerperium
   - (ii) Hyperthyroidism, hypothyroidism, hypoadrenalism, acromegaly
   - (iii) Haemochromatosis, glycogen storage disease (Pompe's), gargoylism (Hurler's), porphyria
   - (iv) Thiamine deficiency (beri-beri)
   - (v) Amyloidosis
3. *Neuromuscular*
   - (i) Muscular dystrophy, especially Duchenne's and dystrophia myotonica
   - (ii) Friedreich's ataxia
4. *Vasculitis* (including Löffler's disease)
5. *Leukaemia or granulomatous infiltrate (sarcoidosis)*
6. *Allergic,* e.g. serum sickness
7. *Drugs and chemicals*
   - (i) Metals—cobalt, antimony, arsenic
   - (ii) Alcohol
   - (iii) Emetine
   - (iv) Phenothiazine and tricyclic antidepressants
   - (v) Anaesthetics
8. *Radiation*

COMPLICATIONS OF MYOCARDIAL INFARCTION

1. Cardiac arrhythmia: Almost any, but particularly—
   - (i) Sinus bradycardia often with nodal escape
   - (ii) Supraventricular tachycardia, atrial flutter, atrial fibrillation
   - (iii) Ventricular tachycardia, flutter or fibrillation
   - (iv) Heart block (all degrees)
   - (v) Cardiac asystole
2. LVF
3. Hypotension and 'shock'
4. Pulmonary embolism (usually from leg veins)
5. Mural thrombus and systemic emboli
6. Pericarditis
7. Ruptured papillary muscle (causing mitral regurgitation)
8. VSD
9. Cardiac aneurysm or rupture
10. Dressler's syndrome (with late onset pleuropericarditis)
11. Frozen shoulder and 'shoulder hand' syndrome
12. Iatrogenic; drugs, pacing, etc.
13. Psychological, including 'L chest pain' and psychosexual problems
14. Psychiatric, including depression and paranoia
15. Social, e.g. loss of job and driving licence

CAUSES OF SYNCOPE

(Transient loss of consciousness, usually due to inadequate cerebral blood flow or hypoxaemia)

1. **Vasovagal**
   - (i) Emotion, heat, standing still
   - (ii) Loss of blood or plasma, dehydration
   - (iii) Carotid sinus hypersensitivity
   - (iv) Postural hypotension
       Prolonged recumbency
       Vasodilator drugs
       Autonomic neuropathy: diabetes, Riley–Day, Shy–Drager (see pp. 130, 131), etc.
       Micturition syncope

2. **Cardiac**
   - (i) Cardiac standstill—vagal inhibition
   - (ii) Stokes–Adams (heart block)
   - (iii) Ventricular tachycardia or fibrillation
   - (iv) Aortic stenosis, hypertrophic cardiomyopathy
   - (v) Cyanotic cong. heart disease (fall in Po_2)
   - (vi) Cough syncope (obstructed venous return)
   - (vii) Massive pulmonary embolism

(viii)   Massive haemopericardium
(ix)   Atrial myxoma, ball-valve thrombus
(x)   Cardiogenic 'shock' (myocardial infarct)

3. Vascular defect
  (i)   Carotid or vertebrobasilar insufficiency
     Atheroma, thrombosis, embolism
     Migraine
     Cervical spondylosis, strangulation, etc.
  (ii)   Subclavian steal syndrome

4. Hypoxaemia
e.g. high altitude, anaemia
For other causes of coma, see page 101

CARDIAC ARREST

Causes
1. Myocardial ischaemia
2. Hypoxia (e.g. in anaesthesia)
3. Vagal reflexes (e.g. carotid sinus)
4. Hyperkalaemia
5. Hypothermia
6. Hypercapnia
7. Electrocution
8. Drugs, e.g. digitalis, quinidine, adrenaline
9. Diagnostic procedures (cardiac catheterization, bronchoscopy, etc.)
10. Severe hypotension
11. Massive pulmonary embolism

'SHOCK'

Clinical shock may be defined as a syndrome where inadequate blood supply and elimination of tissue metabolites lead to functional and/or structural disturbances in essential organs

Causes of clinical shock
1. *Hypovolaemia*
   Haemorrhage, trauma, dehydration, burns
2. *Cardiac failure*
  (i)   Pump failure
  (ii)   Arrhythmia
  (iii)   Obstruction (e.g. pulmonary embolism)
3. *Sepsis*
4. *Anaphylaxis*

CAUSES OF PERICARDITIS
1. Infective
   (i) Viral
   (ii) Bacterial (pyogenic or TB)
   (iii) Fungal
   (iv) Parasitic
2. Rheumatic fever
3. Collagen-vascular, especially SLE
4. Cardiovascular
   (i) Myocardial infarction
   (ii) Postinfarction syndrome
   (iii) Postcardiotomy syndrome
   (iv) Aortic dissection
   (v) Endomyocardial fibrosis
5. Neoplasm, especially bronchial carcinoma
6. Metabolic
   (i) Uraemia
   (ii) Hypothyroidism
   (iii) Hyperuricaemia
7. Trauma
8. Drugs (phenylbutazone, procainamide, hydrallazine, practalol)
9. Radiation
10. Idiopathic (probably viral)

ARTERIAL HYPERTENSION

Causes of pulmonary hypertension
1. *Passive*
   Secondary to raised L atrial pressure (MS or LVF)
2. *Hyperdynamic*
   L to R shunt (ASD, VSD, PDA and TAPVD)
3. *Reactive*
   (i) Vasoconstriction secondary to hypoxia
       High altitude
       Chronic bronchitis
       Kyphoscoliosis
       Upper respiratory tract obstruction
       Respiratory depression
   (ii) Obstructive
       Pulmonary thrombi or emboli
       Arteritis
       Parasites, e.g. schistosomiasis
4. *Drugs,* e.g. fenfluramine

Causes of systemic hypertension
A *Essential*
B *Secondary*
  1. Renal
      (i) Ischaemia (esp. renal artery stenosis)
      (ii) Diffuse renal disease
  2. Hormonal
      (i) Phaeochromocytoma
      (ii) Cushing's
      (iii) Oral contraceptives (increase angiotensin precursor)
      (iv) Primary aldosteronism (Conn's)
      (v) Acromegaly
  3. Coarctation
  4. Drugs (q.v.)
  5. Polycythaemia vera
  6. Toxaemia of pregnancy
  7. Prolonged alcoholism
  8. Neurogenic, e.g. head injury
  9. Acute intermittent porphyria
  10. Endothelioma (v. rare)

Drugs which may induce systemic hypertension
  1. Oestrogens and oral contraceptives
  2. Corticosteroids
  3. Cyclosporin
  4. Sympathomimetics (e.g. phenylpropranolamine in 'cold cures')
  5. Carbenoxolone, liquorice
  6. Clonidine overdose or withdrawal
  7. Erythropoietin
  8. Drug interactions, e.g. guanethidine with tricyclic
      antidepressants or indomethacin or methylamphetamine

ELECTROCARDIOGRAPHY

Cardiac axis

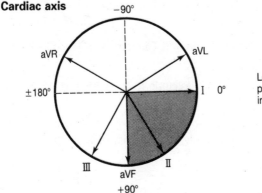

Leads with the maximum positive deflection indicate the cardiac axis

Normal axis is 0° to + 90°
Right axis deviation is + 90° to + 180°
Left axis deviation is 0° to – 120°
(But axis of 0° to – 30° may occur in stocky build, pregnancy and ascites)

Ventricular hypertrophy

Minimal criteria for LVH
Either R in aVL > 13 mm
Or R in V5 or 6 > 27 mm
Or S in V1 + R in V5 or 6 > 35 mm, providing the circulation is not hyperdynamic

Minimal criteria for RVH
Rs or qR complex in V1 or V3r with ventricular activation time > 0.03 sec, QRS < 0.12 sec, and axis deviation

Combined LVH and RVH
Signs of LVH in precordial leads with a frontal plane axis of more than + 90°

R wave predominance in V1–V2
RVH
RBBB
Posterior myocardial infarction
Hypertrophic cardiomyopathy
WPW syndrome (Type A)

ECG signs of infarction
1. *Antero-septal*
Pathological Q and/or ST elevation and T inversion in leads I, aVL and V1–4
2. *Antero-lateral*
Pathological Q and/or ST elevation and T inversion in leads I, aVL and V4–6
3. *Inferior (diaphragmatic)*
Pathological Q and/or ST elevation and T inversion in leads II, III and aVF
4. *True posterior*
Tall R waves in leads V1 and V2. (Exclude RVH, RBBB and Wolff–Parkinson–White)
5. *Subendocardial*
ST depression and T inversion in overlying leads, with reciprocal ST elevation and upright T in leads from the opposite surface and in cavity leads

Causes of low T waves
1. Thick chest wall or emphysema
2. Pericardial effusion
3. Ischaemia
4. Myocarditis or cardiomyopathy
5. Constrictive pericarditis
6. Hypothyroidism, hypopituitarism or hypoadrenalism
7. Nonpenetrating chest trauma
8. Drugs—digitalis, quinidine
9. Hypokalaemia or hypocalcaemia
10. Abdominal visceral disease, e.g. pancreatitis, cholecystitis
11. Post-tachycardia
12. Physiological
    (i)   Juvenile pattern (esp. in Negroes)
    (ii) Eating a large meal or swallowing ice
    (iii) Anxiety
    (iv) Delirium tremens
    (v)   Hyperventilation

Causes of LBBB
1. Ischaemic heart disease
2. Hypertension
3. Aortic valve disease
4. Cardiomyopathy
5. Myocarditis
6. Conduction system fibrosis

Causes of RBBB
1. Normal (especially in young people)
2. RV strain (especially pulmonary embolism)
3. ASD (especially ostium secundum), Fallot's tetralogy, pulmonary stenosis
4. Myocardial ischaemia
5. Myocarditis
6. Drugs—class 1a anti-arrhythmics
7. Hyperkalaemia

ECG changes of hyperkalaemia
Tall T
Prolonged PR
Flattened P
Wide QRS
May be ventricular tachycardia or fibrillation

ECG changes of hypokalaemia
Flattened T
Prolonged PR
Depressed ST
Tall U

Hypercalcaemia: shortens QT
HyPOcalcaemia: PrOlongs QT

Causes of prolonged QT interval

Hereditary
Romano–Ward
Jervell–Lange–Nielsen

Drugs
Amiodarone
Pimozide
Terfenadine
Astemizole
Tricyclics
Vaughan-Williams class Ia and III anti-arrhythmics

Metabolic
Hypocalcaemia
Hypokalaemia
Hyperventilation

Others
Acute myocardial infarction
Prolonged parenteral nutrition
Mitral valve prolapse
Organic insecticide poisoning
Alcoholic liver disease

ECG in pulmonary embolism
Sinus tachycardia
Right axis deviation
Dominant R wave in lead V1
Right bundle branch block
T wave inversion V1–V3
S wave in V6

Supraventricular tachycardia versus ventricular tachycardia
Ventricular tachycardia more likely if—
   Broad complex QRS
   AV dissociation   Variable 1st heart sound
                           Intermittent cannon waves
                           Capture or fusion beats
   Bifid upright QRS—Taller 1st peak in V1
   Deep S wave in V6
   Concordant QRS in V1–V6

CARDIAC CATHETERIZATION—Normal values

	Pressure (mmHg)	
R atrium	−1.5 to zero	
R ventricle	18/0 to 2	
Pulmonary artery	18/8	
Pulmonary 'wedge'	4	
L atrium	4	
L ventricle	130/0 to 10	
Oxygen saturation of mixed venous blood (PA)		65–75%
Oxygen saturation of systemic arterial blood		96–98%

Chest disease

LUNG ANATOMY

BRONCHOPULMONARY SEGMENTS

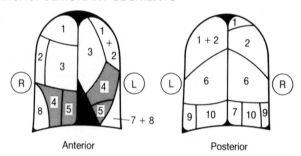

Anterior   Posterior

Right lung
Upper lobe
1. Apical
2. Posterior
3. Anterior

Middle lobe
4. Lateral
5. Medial

Lower lobe
6. Apical
7. Medial basal
8. Anterior basal
9. Lateral basal
10. Posterior basal

Left lung
Upper lobe
1 & 2. Apico-posterior
3. Anterior
4. Superior lingular
5. Inferior lingular

Lower lobe
6. Apical
7 & 8. Antero-medial basal
9. Lateral basal
10. Posterior basal

LUNG MARKINGS

Upper border of lower lobe (oblique fissure). 2nd thoracic spine posteriorly to 6th rib in mammary line
Upper border of (R) middle lobe (transverse fissure). Horizontal line from 4th rib at sternum to the above line
Inferior border of lungs. 8th rib in midaxillary line

PHYSIOLOGY

SPIROMETRY

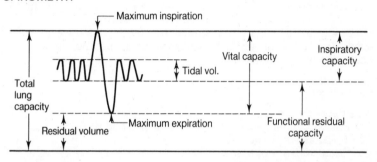

The resting expiratory level is the most constant reference point on the spirometer tracing

Minute ventilation
Product of tidal volume and number of respirations per minute

Vital capacity
Largest volume a subject can expire after a single maximal inspiration. Normal values increase with size of subject and decrease with age (about 4.5 litres in young adult male). Can be reduced in practically any lung or chest wall disease

Forced vital capacity (FVC)
The vital capacity when the expiration is performed as rapidly as possible

FEV$_1$ (Forced expiratory volume in one second)
Volume expired during first second of FVC
Ratio $\dfrac{FEV_1}{FVC}$ should be 75% or more, and is reduced in obstructive airway diseases (asthma, emphysema, bronchitis)

Peak flow
Maximum expiratory flow rate achieved during a forced expiration. A convenient way to detect a reduction in ventilatory function. Also

useful for serial measurements in the same patient and for assessing response to bronchial antispasmodics

Residual volume
Obtained by subtracting expiratory reserve volume from functional residual capacity. Residual volume is normally 20 to 25% of total lung capacity but increases in elderly, and in overinflation of the lungs (emphysema, asthma)

Anatomical dead space
The volume of air in the mouth, pharynx, trachea and bronchi up to the terminal bronchioles (about 150 ml). In disease the physiological dead space may greatly exceed the anatomical dead space due to disorders of the ventilation/perfusion ratio, but in health the two are identical

DIFFUSION

Rate depends on:
1. Pressure difference between alveolar gas and RBC
2. Thickness of tissue
3. Characteristics of tissue
4. Available surface area

Diffusion defects
Carbon dioxide is about 20 times more diffusible than oxygen. In diffusion defects the *arterial* Po_2 is normal or slightly reduced at rest, but decreases markedly after exercise due to increased tissue uptake of O_2. *Arterial* Pco_2 is normal or even reduced at rest (due to hyperventilation) and tends to fall on exercise

Diffusing capacity
Expressed as ml/min/mmHg pressure difference (or mmol/min/kPa)
May be *reduced* in:
1. Alveolocapillary block
    (i)   pulmonary oedema
    (ii) pulmonary fibrosis
    (iii) infiltrative lesions, e.g. sarcoidosis and lymphangitis carcinomatosa
2. Reduction in area available for diffusion
    (i)   emphysema
    (ii) multiple pulmonary emboli
    (iii) pneumonectomy, cysts, etc.
3. Anaemia
May be *increased* in:
1. Increased pulmonary capillary bed
2. Polycythaemia

Compliance

The volume change produced by unit change of pressure, expressed as litres/cm H_2O(or l/kPa)

Pulmonary compliance
A measure of lung elasticity. It is reduced when the lungs are abnormally stiff due to pulmonary venous congestion or infiltrative or fibrotic lesions of the lungs. It is increased in emphysema

Thoracic cage compliance
Decreased in kyphoscoliosis, skeletal muscle spasticity and pectus excavatum

BLOOD-GAS ANALYSIS

These values must be related to the normal levels expected for the subject, e.g. baby, old man, pregnant woman

Hypoxia
Oxygen deficiency at a specified site

Hypoxaemia
Oxygen deficiency in the blood. In arterial blood of normal resting adult
P_{CO_2} is about 40 mmHg (4 to 6 kPa)
P_{O_2} is about 90 to 100 mmHg (12 to 15 kPa)

Causes of hypoxaemia
1. Cardiorespiratory disorders
    (i)   Hypoventilation (q.v.)
    (ii) Abnormality of ventilation/perfusion ratio
    (iii) Impaired diffusion
    (iv) Venous to arterial shunt
2. Decreased P_{O_2} of inspired gas, e.g. high altitude
3. Reduction in active haemoglobin, e.g. coal gas poisoning

Causes of hypoventilation
1. Respiratory centre depression
    (i)   Drugs
    (ii) Anoxia
    (iii) Hypercapnia
    (iv) Trauma
    (v)   Raised IC pressure
    (vi) Primary alveolar hypoventilation
          (Pickwickian syndrome, with obesity and hypoventilation)
2. Neural or neuromuscular cause
3. Respiratory muscle disease

4. Limited thoracic movement
   (i) Kyphoscoliosis
   (ii) Elevated diaphragm
5. Limited lung movement
   (i) Pleural effusion
   (ii) Pneumothorax
6. Lung disease
   (i) Obstruction in upper or lower respiratory tract
   (ii) Atelectasis, pneumonia, etc.

Causes of hyperventilation
1. Anxiety, hysteria, pain
2. CNS lesions: meningitis, encephalitis, trauma, CVA, etc.
3. Drugs: salicylates, analeptics, adrenaline
4. Increased metabolism: hyperthyroidism, fever, etc.
5. Anoxia
6. Metabolic acidosis
7. Pulmonary reflexes: irritant gases, pneumothorax, atelectasis, left ventricular failure
8. Hypotension
9. Artificial ventilation

Cheyne–Stokes respiration
Normal in infancy

Short cycle   Neurological lesion
                 (pons or medulla)

Long cycle   Opiates
                 Renal failure
                 Pneumonia
                 Heart failure
                 Cerebral vascular disease

PHYSICAL SIGNS

CRACKLES AND WHEEZES

Crackles
Crackles (formerly called râles, moist sounds or crepitations) are nonmusical lung sounds of short duration. Inspiratory crackles are produced by abrupt opening of closed airways in regions of the lung deflated to residual volume. Early inspiratory crackles are associated with severe airways obstruction, late inspiratory crackles with a restrictive defect due to fibrosis, infiltration or oedema
   Friction between the two layers of the pleura can also produce crackles, but they are usually louder, localized and occur in expiration as well as inspiration

Wheezes
Wheezes (formerly called rhonchi) are musical lung sounds produced by air passing at high velocity through an airway narrowed to the point of closure. The pitch of the wheeze is determined by the velocity of the air-jet and is independent of the calibre and length of the airway. Thus in severe airway obstruction wheeze may be absent if ventilation is so reduced that the air-jet slows below the critical minimum velocity

SIGNS OF DIFFUSE AIRWAYS OBSTRUCTION WITH LUNG DISTENSION

1. **Inspection**
   (i) Increased AP diameter of chest
   (ii) Excavation of supraclavicular fossae during inspiration
   (iii) Jugular venous filling during expiration

2. **Palpation**
   (i) Decreased length of trachea above sternal notch
   (ii) Tracheal descent with inspiration
   (iii) Use of accessory muscles
   (iv) Loss of bucket-handle movement of upper ribs
   (v) Paradoxical movement of costal margin

3. **Percussion**
   (i) Decreased heart and liver dullness

4. **Auscultation**
   (i) Diminished breath sounds
   (ii) Forced expiratory time exceeds 4 seconds

EMPHYSEMA

Definition: Enlargement of the air-spaces distal to the terminal bronchioles, either from dilatation or destruction of their walls. Some authorities (e.g. WHO and American Thoracic Society) restrict the term to conditions accompanied by tissue destruction. Both chest radiology and transfer factor for carbon monoxide are poor indicators of the extent of emphysema, but the CT scan of transverse thoracic sections can be used to quantitate and locate areas of emphysema

CHRONIC BRONCHITIS

Definition: Cough with sputum for at least 3 months in each year for 3 years.

THE EMPHYSEMA–CHRONIC BRONCHITIS SPECTRUM

	Emphysema ('Pink Puffers')	Chronic bronchitis ('Blue Bloaters')
Course	Relentlessly progressive dyspnoea	Intermittent dyspnoea with exacerbations
Sputum	Scanty	Profuse, mucopurulent
Cor pulmonale	Infrequent, usually terminal	Frequent and remittent
Polycythaemia	Uncommon	Common
CXR	Attenuated peripheral vessels	Normal peripheral vessels
Arterial $P\text{CO}_2$	Normal	Raised
Alveolar gas transfer	Reduced	Normal
Nocturnal hypoxaemia	Mild	Profound, especially in REM sleep, and associated with pulmonary hypertension

Most patients have both conditions to a greater or lesser degree, and some authors prefer the term chronic obstructive pulmonary disease (COPD) for the combined condition. Trials have shown that 'continuous' oxygen therapy at home can improve both life expectancy and quality of life in severe COPD. Patients should be considered for this if they have an arterial $P\text{O}_2$ of 55 mmHg or less for 3 weeks when in a stable clinical state, or if they have cor pulmonale and secondary polycythaemia

CAUSES OF EMPHYSEMA

Localized
1. Congenital
2. Compensatory, due to lung collapse, scarring or resection
3. Partial bronchial occlusion
   (i)   foreign body
   (ii) neoplasm
   (iii) peribronchial lymphadenopathy (e.g. TB)
4. Rarely unilateral emphysema due to bronchiolitis before age 8 years (Macleod's syndrome)

Generalized
1. Idiopathic ('primary')
2. Associated with chronic bronchitis, chronic asthma or pneumoconiosis } usually centrilobular
3. Senile (physiological)

4. Familial (some due to α_1-antitrypsin deficiency, when the disease is usually basal)

PATHOGENESIS OF EMPHYSEMA

Cigarette smoke attracts alveolar macrophages to cluster around the small terminal bronchioles, and the macrophages then attract circulating polymorphonuclear neutrophils to the site. These release an elastase which attacks the lung interstitial matrix. The elastase is normally inactivated by a plasma protein, the α_1-protease inhibitor
    Deficiency of the protease inhibitor, also called α_1-antitrypsin (AAT), is associated with the early onset of emphysema (before age 50). Homozygotes for the AAT deficiency gene have the protease inhibitor phenotype PiZZ. The normal phenotype is PiMM, and heterozygotes have PiMZ. The significance of PiMZ is uncertain, but in some studies it appears to increase the risk of emphysema
    Infants with PiZZ may develop cirrhosis and cholestasis. Adults with PiZZ may develop cirrhosis and hepatic cancer

BRONCHIECTASIS

Dilatation of the bronchi, usually accompanied by recurrent bronchial suppuration

Pathogenesis
Increased outward traction on the bronchi and weakness of the bronchial wall due to inflammation are both important

Causes
1. Infection
    (i)   Bronchiolitis of infancy
    (ii) Measles or pertussis in children
    (iii) Post bronchopneumonic collapse in adults
    (iv) Commonly in post-primary TB, but apical, therefore secondary infection is unusual
2. Bronchial stenosis or occlusion
    (i)   Adenoma or carcinoma
    (ii) Foreign body or asthma casts
    (iii) Lymphadenopathy
3. Pulmonary aspergillosis
4. Cystic fibrosis
5. Immotile cilia (Kartagener's)
6. Neuropathic (Chagas')
7. Many cases are idiopathic

CAUSES OF CHRONIC COR PULMONALE

1. Chronic bronchitis or emphysema
2. Chronic asthma
3. Bronchiectasis
4. Pulmonary fibrosis
5. Pulmonary thromboembolism
6. Kyphoscoliosis
7. Chronic neuromuscular disease affecting chest
8. Primary alveolar hypoventilation (including Pickwickian syndrome)

CAUSES OF PERSISTENT COUGH

1. Asthma
2. Bronchiectasis
3. Bronchial carcinoma
4. Chronic bronchitis
5. Infection, e.g. TB
6. Repeated aspiration
7. Severe gastro-oesophageal reflux
8. Pulmonary fibrosis/alveolitis
9. Drugs—especially ACE inhibitors
10. Psychogenic, including habit

HARMFUL EFFECTS OF CIGARETTE SMOKING

1. *Pharmacological effects of nicotine*
    (i) CVS: rise in BP, tachycardia, cutaneous vasoconstriction
    (ii) Autonomic: transient stimulation, followed by depression of all ganglia
    (iii) Increased catecholamines (from adrenal) increase platelet stickiness
    (iv) CNS: stimulation, especially respiratory, vasomotor and emetic centres
    (v) Antidiuretic: due to ADH release
    (vi) Immunological effects: reduction in neutrophil chemotaxis, Ig concentration and NK cell activity
2. *Pharyngeal and bronchial irritation*
    (i) Bronchitis
    (ii) Postoperative pneumonia, etc.
3. *Carcinoma incidence increased*
    (i) Bronchus
    (ii) Oesophagus
    (iii) Prostate
    (iv) Bladder
    NB Synergistic effects, e.g. with asbestos
4. *Cardiovascular disease exacerbated*
    (i) Myocardial ischaemia

(ii) Buerger's
(iii) 'Strokes' (esp. with oral contraceptives)
5. *Peptic ulcer mortality and morbidity increased (delayed healing)* but *not* incidence
6. *Inflammatory bowel disease*
    (i) More frequent relapses in Crohn's
    (ii) Stopping smoking may provoke presentation of ulcerative colitis
7. *Osteoporosis*
8. *Idiosyncrasy*
    (i) Tobacco angina or amblyopia
    (ii) Atrial extrasystoles
    (iii) Hypoglycaemia
    (iv) Polycythaemia
9. *Cirrhosis incidence increased*
    (probably due to associated alcoholism)
10. *Skin*
    (i) Staining of fingers and hair
    (ii) Facial wrinkling enhanced
    (iii) Association with pustular psoriasis
11. *Miscellaneous,* e.g. effects on sperm morphogenesis, impaired memory
12. *Passive smoking effects*
    (i) Effect on fetus
        Smoking during pregnancy restricts fetal growth and increases perinatal mortality rate (including cot-deaths). Physical and mental retardation persists into childhood
    (ii) Effects on non-smokers
        Smoke may provoke cough, asthma, angina. Cancer risk is controversial

INDUSTRIAL CHEST DISEASE

1. *Mineral dust pneumoconiosis*
   Coal dust, silicates (including talc, kaolin and asbestos), iron, tin, tungsten, aluminium, etc.
2. *Disease due to organic dust*
   Byssinosis, farmer's lung, bagassosis, mushroom-worker's lung, paprika-splitter's lung, etc.
3. *Disease due to industrial gases and fumes*
   Manganese pneumonitis, cadmium emphysema, silo-filler's disease, metal fume fever (ZnO), etc.
4. *Occupational lung cancer*
   Nickel-refining, chromate workers, retort-house workers in gasworks, asbestos workers, etc.
5. *Chronic bronchitis*
   Many heavy, dusty industries

COMPLICATIONS OF ASBESTOS INHALATION

1. Pleural plaques (may calcify)
2. Pleural effusion (or rarely acute pleuritis)
3. Asbestosis (diffuse intestitial pulmonary fibrosis)
4. Mesothelioma
   (i)   Malignant (usually caused by crocidolite)
   (ii) Benign (a peripheral solitary lesion)
5. Lung cancer (the risk is greatly enhanced by smoking)
6. Pseudotumour of lung

CAUSES OF PULMONARY FIBROSIS

1. *Infections*
   Especially TB, mycosis, varicella, psittacosis
2. *Pneumoconiosis*
   Inorganic
   Silica, asbestos, talc, kaolin, tungsten, iron, Be, Al, china-clay
   Coal dust, but only in progressive massive fibrosis or Caplan's syndrome
3. *Extrinsic allergic alveolitis*
   Farmers, bird-fanciers, cheese-washers, malt-workers, etc. and bagassosis
4. *Idiopathic (cryptogenic) fibrosing alveolitis* (also called idiopathic pulmonary fibrosis)
5. *Collagen-vascular disease,* including rheumatoid lung
6. *Sarcoidosis*
7. *Aspiration*
   Especially lipoid pneumonitis
8. *Cardiac*
   Pulmonary oedema, mitral stenosis ossification, multiple pulmonary infarcts, 'uraemic lung'
9. *Drugs and poisons*
   Cytotoxic, e.g. busulphan
   Others, e.g. nitrofurantoin, paraquat
10. *Neoplastic*
    Alveolar cell carcinoma, lymphangitis carcinomatosa
11. *Miscellaneous*
    Systemic sclerosis, SLE, radiation, eosinophilic granuloma, tuberous sclerosis (epiloia), xanthomatosis, biliary cirrhosis, hypogammaglobulinaemia
    When shown a chest radiograph with widespread miliary densities, do not offer pneumoconiosis as a first suggestion if breast shadows are visible

DRUG-INDUCED PULMONARY DISEASES

1. *Asthma*	Predictable:	β-blockers
		Cholinergic drugs
		Cholinesterases inhibitors
	Idiosyncratic:	NSAID
		Tartrazine
		Penicillins
		IV iron
2. *ARDS* (p. 35)	Hydrochlorothiazide	
	Isoxsuprine	
3. *Pulmonary eosinophilia*	Sulphonamides	
	Penicillins	
	Sulphasalazine	
	L-tryptophan	
	Nitrofurantoin	
4. *Alveolitis*	Bleomycin	
	Busulphan	
	Nitrofurantoin	
	Amiodarone	
	Methysergide	
5. *Pulmonary oedema*	Heroin	
	Methadone	
6. *Pulmonary hypertension*	Aminorex	
7. *Granulomas*	Methrotrexate	
	Mineral oil	
8. *Pleuritis*	Procainamide	
	Phenytoin	
	Hydrallazine	
9. *Oculomucocutaneous syndrome*	Practolol	

Other drugs have indirect adverse effects on the lungs
1. *Infection* (esp. opportunistic or TB) due to glucocorticoids or cytotoxic drugs
2. *Aspiration,* e.g. due to oversedation
3. *Pulmonary embolism,* e.g. due to thrombophlebitis
4. *Bleeding,* e.g. due to anticoagulants
5. *Vasculitis,* e.g. due to sulphonamides, etc.

CAUSES OF PNEUMOTHORAX

1. **Traumatic**

2. **Iatrogenic**
    (i) Thoracentesis, thoracic or cervical surgery

(ii)   Artificial pneumothorax
(iii) Artificial ventilation

3. **Spontaneous**
   (i)   *Localized air space disorder*
         Congenital bullae
         Localized emphysema
         Acquired cysts, etc.
   (ii) *Generalized emphysema*
   (iii) *Secondary to specific lung disease*
         Diffuse cystic disease
         e.g. congenital cysts, bronchiectasis, eosinophilic
         granuloma, tuberous sclerosis (epiloia)
         TB
         Silicosis
         Lung abscess
         Malignancy
         Hydatid cysts
   (iv) *Secondary to spontaneous mediastinal emphysema*
         Asthma, labour, straining at stool, etc.
         Rapid decompression of divers
   (v)   *Associated with menstruation*
         ? Endometriosis

CAUSES OF PLEURAL EFFUSION

1. *Transudate* (Less than 25 g protein/litre. Implies a systemic
   cause)
   (i)   Cardiac failure
   (ii) Nephrotic syndrome
   (iii) Hepatic failure or abscess
   (iv) Hypothyroidism
2. *Exudate* (More than 25 g protein/litre. Implies a local cause)
   (i)   Pneumonia
   (ii)   Malignancy (bronchial Ca., secondary Ca., lymphoma or
          mesothelioma)
   (iii) TB
   (iv)   Pulmonary infarction
   (v)   Collagen-vascular disease (especially SLE)
   (vi)   Drugs, e.g. cytotoxic drugs, phenylhydantoin, practolol,
          isoniazid, methysergide
   (vii) Benign asbestos disease
   (viii) Post-pericardiectomy or post-myocardial infarct (Dressler's)
   (ix)   Yellow nail syndrome, with primary lymphoedema
   (x)   Subphrenic abscess
   (xi)   Meig's syndrome (with ovarian fibroma)
   (xii) Post-oesophageal rupture

CAUSES OF PULMONARY OEDEMA

1. **Increased capillary pressure**
   (i) Left heart failure
       Atrial, e.g. mitral stenosis
       Ventricular, e.g. hypertension or myocardial infarct
   (ii) Pulmonary venous obstruction
   (iii) Overload of i.v. fluid

2. **Increased capillary permeability**
   (i) Pneumonia (viral, bacterial)
   (ii) Inhaled toxins, e.g. chlorine, mustard gas
   (iii) Circulating toxins, e.g. paraquat, septicaemia, snake
        venoms, histamine
   (iv) Diffuse intravascular coagulation
   (v) Renal failure
   (vi) Radiation pneumonitis
   (vii) 'Shock-lung' (post-traumatic)

3. **Decreased plasma oncotic pressure**
   Hypo-albuminaemia

4. **Lymphatic obstruction**

5. **Unknown mechanism**
   High altitude
   Raised intracranial pressure
   Heroin overdose
   Pulmonary embolism, esp. fat
   Eclampsia

ADULT RESPIRATORY DISTRESS SYNDROME (ARDS)
('Respirator lung')

Various massive insults to the lung can cause injury to the gas
exchange interface, producing dyspnoea, laboured breathing,
noncardiogenic pulmonary oedema and hypoxaemia which is
refractory to oxygen therapy
    The chest X-ray shows a diffuse and rapidly progressive
infiltration which characteristically spares the costophrenic angles
(unlike cardiogenic pulmonary oedema)
    Surfactant abnormalities are thought to be involved in the
pathogenesis

CAUSES OF ARDS

1. 'Shock'
2. Trauma (may be pulmonary or multisystem)

3. Infection (usually overwhelming)
4. Disseminated intravascular coagulation
5. Emboli
     (i) Fat
     (ii) Amniotic fluid
6. Aspiration (esp. gastric contents)
7. Inhaled toxins (smoke, gases)
8. Pancreatitis
9. Massive transfusion
10. Oxygen toxicity
11. Poisons, esp. Paraquat
12. CNS hypoxia
13. Narcotic drug abuse
14. Radiation pneumonitis

CAUSES OF SLOW RESOLUTION OF PNEUMONIA

1. Bronchial obstruction
   Neoplasm, foreign body (especially peanut), etc.
2. Inappropriate chemotherapy
   Especially for stapylococcus, klebsiella, TB, mycosis
3. Decreased host resistance
   Cachexia, agranulocytosis, immunoglobulin defects, LVF, etc.
   NB *AIDS patients*
4. Pharyngeal pouch with 'spilling'
5. Formation of abscess, empyema or serous effusion
6. Other causes of pulmonary fibrosis (p. 32)

PULMONARY MANIFESTATIONS OF AIDS

1. **Opportunistic infections**
     (i)   *Pneumocystis carinii*
     (ii) *Cytomegalovirus*
     (iii) *Mycobact. avium*-complex
     (iv) *Cryptococcus neoformans*
     (v)   *Nocardia*
     (vi) *Fungi*

2. **Non-opportunistic infections**
e.g. Tuberculosis, histoplasmosis or coccidioidomycosis

3. **Kaposi's sarcoma of the lungs**

4. **Lymphoma of lung**

5. **Lymphocytic interstitial pneumonitis**

PNEUMONIA

Indicators of increased risk of mortality—

1. **Clinical**
   > 60 years old
   Respiratory rate > 30/min
   Low diastolic BP < 60 mmHg
   Atrial fibrillation
   Acute confusion
   Immunosuppression

2. **Investigations**
   Raised blood urea
   Low WBC
   Very high WBC
   Low albumin
   Low Pao_2 < 8 kPa

CAUSES OF LUNG ABSCESS

1. **Malignancy**
   (i)   Necrotic bronchial carcinoma
   (ii) Secondary to bronchial obstruction
   (iii) Spill-over of pus or slough

2. **Aspiration**
   (i)   Oral or pharyngeal sepsis
   (ii) Pharyngeal pouch
   (iii) Oesophageal obstruction, tracheo-oesophageal fistula
   (iv) Drowning
   (v)   Bronchiectasis elsewhere in lung
   (vi) Coma, anaesthesia, alcoholic debauch, etc.

3. **Vascular embolus**
   (i)   Secondary infection of pulmonary infarct
   (ii) Septic emboli due to pyaemia

4. **Specific abscesses**
   (i)   Staphylococcal
   (ii) Friedlander's (klebsiella)
   (iii) TB
   (iv) Actinomycosis and other fungi
   (v)   *Entamoeba histolytica*

5. **Bronchial obstruction**
   Benign tumour, foreign body, mucoviscidosis, etc.

6. **Infection of congenital or acquired cysts**

LUNG DISEASE CAUSED BY ASPERGILLUS

1. Asthma
2. Extrinsic allergic alveolitis (e.g. in maltworkers)
3. Aspergilloma
4. Invasive aspergillosis
5. Bronchopulmonary eosinophilia (q.v.)

Bronchopulmonary eosinophilia
1. *Eosinophilic bronchitis*
    (i) Uncomplicated asthma
    (ii) Asthma with casts, partial collapse and Aspergillus hypersensitivity
    (iii) As (ii), but with no Aspergillus hypersensitivity
2. *Eosinophilic pneumonia*
    (i) Parasitic, e.g. Ascaris (localized) or microfilariae (diffuse)
    (ii) Fungal, e.g. Aspergillus infection
    (iii) Drugs, e.g. nitrofurantoin, PAS, phenylbutazone
    (iv) Occupational, e.g. epoxy resins
    (v) Idiopathic ('prolonged pulmonary eosinophilia')
NB Polyarteritis nodosa is now regarded as a separate entity

COMPLICATIONS OF CA. BRONCHUS

1. **Local effects**
    (i) Bronchial obstruction
        Collapse
        Pneumonia
        Abscess
        Emphysema
    (ii) SV caval obstruction
    (iii) Pulmonary artery or vein compression
    (iv) Cervical sympathetic, recurrent laryngeal or phrenic nerve invasion
    (v) Pleural effusion, empyema
    (vi) Direct spread into mediastinum, chest wall, brachial plexus, etc.
    (vii) Erosion of large vessel

2. **Metastases**
Hilar nodes, liver, cerebrum, adrenals, bone

3. **Non-metastatic extrapulmonary effects**
    (i) Cachexia, anaemia, etc.
    (ii) Hypertrophic pulmonary osteoarthropathy and clubbing
    (iii) Neuropathy or myopathy (p. 129)
    (iv) Skin lesions (p. 196)
    (v) Ectopic humoral syndromes (p. 157)

Small cell (oat cell) carcinoma accounts for 25% of all lung cancer. It disseminates early, but is relatively sensitive to combination chemotherapy. It arises from endocrine cells of the APUD-system, and may secrete various polypeptide hormones, particularly *bombesin*

NB *Polycythaemia* very rarely occurs with bronchial carcinoma, but may occur with renal carcinoma etc. (p. 86)

HYPERTROPHIC OSTEOARTHROPATHY

A triad comprising
1. Clubbing
2. Periosteal new bone formation
3. Arthritis

CAUSES

1. **Thoracic**
   (i) Pulmonary neoplasm (Ca., mesothelioma)
   (ii) Chronic pulmonary suppuration
   (iii) Fibrosing alveolitis
   (iv) Mediastinal tumours
   (v) Asbestosis

2. **Cardiovascular**
   (i) Bacterial endocarditis
   (ii) Cyanotic congenital heart disease
   (iii) Atrial myxoma
   (iv) Arteriovenous fistula

3. **Extrathoracic lesions**
   (i) Gastroenterological
       Cirrhosis (esp. biliary)
       Ulcerative colitis
       Crohn's disease
       Coeliac disease
   (ii) Thyrotoxicosis (thyroid acropachy)
   (iii) Rarely   Dysproteinaemia (esp. alpha chain disease)
                  Pyelonephritis
                  Syphilis
                  Pregnancy

4. **Congenital** *(Pachydermoperiostosis)*
The syndrome may be only partially expressed, e.g. congenital clubbing

Possible pathogenetic factors in clubbing
1. Megakaryocytes reaching the fingertips and releasing platelet-derived growth factor
2. Increased autonomic activity (stimulation of afferent tracts of the vagus)

MEDIASTINAL MASSES

Causes
1. *Lymphadenopathy*
   Lymphoma, sarcoidosis, infection (especially TB), carcinoma metastasis
2. *Aorta*
   Unfolding, aneurysm, coarctation
3. *Oesophagus*
   Corkscrew oesophagus (congenital elongation), megaoesophagus (achalasia), enterogenous cyst, neoplasm
4. *Retrosternal goitre*
5. *Cysts*
   Dermoid, teratoma, pericardial 'spring-water' cysts, hydatid, bronchial cyst
6. *Thymoma*
7. *Herniae*
   Hiatus hernia, diaphragmatic hernia, lung herniation
8. *Neurogenic*
   Neurilemmoma, neurofibroma, sympathetic ganglioneuroma, sympathetic neuroblastoma
9. *Miscellaneous rare causes*
   Cardiac aneurysm or tumour, mesothelioma, lipoma, etc.

Common sites of mediastinal tumours

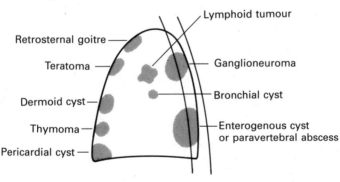

L Lateral view

THE 'NORMAL' CHEST X-RAY

Faced in an exam with a chest X-ray which at first sight appears normal, look for the following:

Apices
1. Small apical pneumothorax
2. Pancoast's tumour

Behind the heart
1. Hiatus hernia
2. Neural tumour
3. Vertebral disease

The heart
1. Valve calcification
2. Slight 'mitralisation' of the heart

Skeletal defects
1. Cervical rib
2. Secondary deposits

Gas
1. Under the diaphragm (beware the post-op. CXR)
2. Pneumomediastinum

Breast shadows
Unilateral mastectomy

Lung anatomy
Azygos lobe

Causes of bilateral hilar lymphadenopathy
Sarcoidosis
Tuberculosis
Lymphoma
Carcinoma
Berylliosis
Histoplasmosis
Coccidioidomycosis
Leukaemia

Causes of upper zone shadowing
Tuberculosis
Sarcoidosis
Ankylosing spondylitis
Extrinsic allergic alveolitis
Aspergillosis
Silicosis
Post-radiation therapy

Gastroenterology

CAUSES OF STOMATITIS

1. *Debilitation, smoking, alcoholism*
2. *Aphthous ulcers*
3. *Infection*
    (i) Viral
          Herpes simplex
          Herpangina
          Hand, foot and mouth disease (coxsackie)
    (ii) Bacterial
          Pyorrhoea and alveolar abscess
          Vincent's angina, TB, syphilis
    (iii) Fungal, especially *Candida*
4. *Associated with systemic disease*
    (i) Behcet's, Reiter's, Stevens–Johnson
    (ii) Leukaemia
    (iii) Neutropenia
    (iv) Crohn's (oral)
    (v) Fe deficiency
    (vi) Vitamin deficiency
          B complex, including B_{12} and folate
    (vii) Cancrum oris (malnutrition, malaria, etc.)
5. *Associated with skin disease*
    (i) Pemphigus vulgaris
    (ii) Benign pemphigoid of mucous membranes
    (iii) Lichen planus
6. *Stomatitis medicamentosa*
    (i) Cytotoxic drugs
    (ii) Bi, Hg, As, Au
    (iii) Antibiotics
7. *Leukoplakia* (**NB** Oral hairy leukoplakia in AIDS)
8. *Neoplasm*
9. *Allergy*
    e.g. dentures and dental medicaments
10. *Caustics and trauma*
    e.g. cheek-biting and dentures

Systemic causes of gingival swelling
1. Pregnancy and oral contraceptives
2. Leukaemia (especially monocytic)
3. Phenytoin
4. Scurvy
5. Heavy metals (especially Hg and As)

CAUSES OF PAROTID GLAND ENLARGEMENT

1. **Infections**
   (i) Viral (mumps, cytomegalic inclusion disease)
   (ii) Bacterial, especially in dehydrated patients

2. **Neoplasia**

3. **Duct blockage**
   e.g. by calculus

4. **Systemic disease**
   (i)   Sjögren's syndrome
   (ii)   Sarcoidosis
   (iii) Drugs (iodides, thiouracil, phenylbutazone, lead)
   (iv)   Cirrhosis
   (v)   Cystic fibrosis
   (vi)   Alcoholism
   (vii) Bulimia
   (viii) Rarely—hyperlipidaemia, malnutrition or vitamin
          deficiency, pregnancy, diabetes mellitus

CAUSES OF DYSPHAGIA

1. **Mouth and pharynx**
   Stomatitis and glossitis
   Oral tumour
   Tonsillitis
   Quinsy, retropharyngeal abscess
   Lymphoma of tonsil

2. **Extrinsic compression of oesophagus or pharynx**
   Neck tumours
   Mediastinal tumours, glands, aneurysm, L atrial enlargement,
   etc.
   Pericardial effusion
   Bronchial carcinoma

3. **Intrinsic disease of oesophagus or pharynx**
   Oesophagitis
   Oesophageal dysmotility
   Cricopharyngeal achalasia

Oesophageal achalasia
Plummer–Vinson syndrome (Paterson–Kelly–Brown)
   (Fe def., glossitis, pharyngeal web and koilonychia)
Pharyngeal pouch
Peptic stricture
Neoplasm
Systemic sclerosis
Chagas' disease (trypanosomiasis)

4. **Foreign body**
   Within the lumen of oesophagus or pharynx

5. **CNS lesions**
   Bulbar and pseudobulbar palsy
   Parkinson's disease
   Muscular dystrophy
   Motor neurone disease
   Myasthenia gravis
   Diphtheritic neuritis

6. **Psychological (globus hystericus)**

RISK FACTORS FOR OESOPHAGEAL MALIGNANCY

Smoking
Alcohol
Barrett's oesophagus
Plummer–Vinson syndrome
Achalasia
Coeliac disease
Previous scars from corrosive ingestion
Familial tylosis

CONTROL OF GASTRIC ACID SECRETION

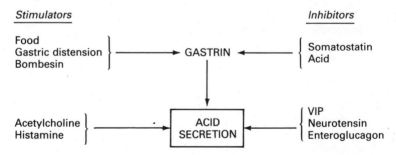

Omeprazole controls gastric acid secretion by irreversibly inhibiting
H^+/K^+ ATPase (proton pump) on the parietal cell

CAUSES OF HYPERGASTRINAEMIA

1. Gastrinoma
2. Antral G-cell hyperplasia
3. Renal failure
4. Achlorhydria
5. Retained and isolated antrum
6. Vagotomy
7. Short bowel syndrome
8. H_2 blockers
9. Omeprazole

CAUSES OF VOMITING

1. **Feeding upsets (in infancy) and dietary indiscretions**

2. **GI irritation**
   Poisons (especially food poisoning)
   Gastritis (especially alcohol-induced)
   Gastric ulcer
   Enteritis (including viral, e.g. Norwalk)

3. **Obstruction**
   Atresia
   Stricture (including malignancy) or stenosis
   Intussusception
   Volvulus
   Strangulated hernia
   Paralytic ileus

4. **Acute intra-abdominal inflammation**
   Hepatitis
   Pancreatitis
   Appendicitis
   Pyelonephritis
   Cholecystitis

5. **Metabolic and endocrine**
   Diabetic precoma
   Pregnancy
   Uraemia
   Hypoadrenalism

6. **CNS**
   Psychogenic
   Severe pain
   Drugs (e.g. digoxin)
   Migraine
   Motion sickness

Meningitis
Menière's, labyrinthitis
Raised intracranial pressure

7. **Miscellaneous**
   Fevers, e.g. pertussis
   Acute dilatation of stomach
   Cyclical vomiting
   Anorexia/bulimia
   Radiation sickness

CAUSES OF HYPOCHLORHYDRIA

1. Pernicious anaemia
2. Gastric ulcer
3. Gastric carcinoma
4. Gastric polyposis
5. Surgery
   (i) Vagotomy
   (ii) Subtotal gastrectomy
6. Iron deficiency
7. Pregnancy
8. Atrophic gastritis (*Helicobacter pylori*)
9. Old age or debility
10. Vitamin deficiency (pellagra)
11. Radiation

RISK FACTORS FOR GASTRIC CANCER

1. Smoking
2. Lower socio-economic class
3. Blood group A
4. Pernicious anaemia
5. Post-gastrectomy
6. *Helicobacter pylori* infection
7. Diet ? nitrosamines
8. Ethnic origin (increased incidence in Japanese)

CAUSES OF HAEMATEMESIS

1. Peptic ulcer
2. Oesophageal varices
3. Erosive gastritis (aspirin, alcohol, etc.)
4. Oesophagitis
5. Mallory–Weiss syndrome (oesophageal tear)
6. Swallowed blood (post-nose bleed)
7. Gastric neoplasm
8. Blood dyscrasia
9. Dieulafoy's abnormality (vascular malformation)

10. Antral vascular ectasia (watermelon stomach)
11. Hereditary haemorrhagic telangiectasia (Osler–Weber–Rendu)
12. Pseudoxanthoma elasticum
13. Ehlers–Danlos syndrome (Cutis hyperelastica)
14. Idiopathic

PEPTIC ULCER

Indications for surgical treatment of peptic ulcer
Acute
(i)   Continuing or life-threatening haemorrhage
      > 4 units if over 60 years
      > 8 units if under 60 years
(ii) Active bleeding not responsive to endoscopic intervention
(iii) Perforation
Chronic
(i)   Pyloric stenosis
(ii) Failure to heal despite adequate acid suppression
(iii) Frequent relapse despite eradication of *Helicobacter pylori*

Side effects of vagotomy
1. Atony of stomach with dilatation
2. Belching and 'bilious' feeling
3. Abdominal distension
4. Diarrhoea
5. Cardiospasm
6. Dysphagia

Medical complications of gastrectomy
1. Calorie deficiency
2. Stomal ulcer or fistula
3. 'Dumping syndrome' (due to jejunal distension)
4. Late 'dumping' (due to hypoglycaemia)
5. Bilious vomiting, distension
6. Postprandial diarrhoea
7. Malabsorption
8. Anaemia (deficiency of Fe, B_{12} or folate)
9. Osteomalacia
10. Hypoanabolic hypoproteinaemia
11. Increased risk of carcinoma in gastric remnant (x4)
12. Recrudescence of pulmonary TB
13. Reflux oesophagitis

MEDICAL CAUSES OF ACUTE ABDOMINAL PAIN

Common causes
1. Food poisoning or dietary indiscretion
2. Peptic ulcer, gastritis, oesophagitis

3. Biliary colic or cholecystitis
4. Pancreatitis
5. Hepatic congestion (hepatitis, cardiac failure)
6. Renal colic, pyelonephritis or cystitis
7. Diverticulitis, ulcerative colitis, Crohn's disease
8. Mesenteric adenitis (children)
9. Mesenteric ischaemia (q.v.)
10. Aortic dissection
11. Gynaecological, e.g.
    Mittelschmerz (ovulation)
    Dysmenorrhoea
    Salpingitis
    Threatened abortion
12. Pain referred from spine or chest (e.g. myocardial infarct)

Less common causes
1. Gastric dilatation, esp. in diabetic ketosis
2. Diaphragmatic pleurisy
3. Herpes zoster
4. Migraine
5. Epilepsy
6. Lead poisoning
7. Tabes dorsalis
8. Acute intermittent porphyria
9. Addison's disease
10. Haemochromatosis
11. Haemolytic crisis (especially sickle-cell anaemia)
12. Haemorrhage into gut wall (e.g. in bleeding disease)
13. Henoch–Schönlein purpura
14. Hepatoma
15. Hypercalcaemia
16. Hyperlipidaemia
17. Uraemia
18. Intestinal parasites
19. Hereditary angio-oedema

Acute small bowel ischaemia

Causes
1. Thrombosis of superior mesenteric artery (e.g. due to atheroma, thrombophilia or oestrogens)
2. Embolism of superior mesenteric artery (e.g. secondary to myocardial infarct)
3. Low-flow non-occlusive states
    (i) Narrowing of superior mesenteric artery trunk
    (ii) Splanchnic vasoconstriction (e.g. digoxin overdose)
    (iii) Low cardiac output
    (iv) Haemoconcentration

Classical features
  (i)   Abrupt onset of severe abdominal pain
  (ii) Paradoxical absence of abdominal signs
  (iii) Rapid onset of hypovolaemic shock

Chronic small bowel ischaemia
Defined as a reduction of the post-prandial intestinal blood flow
sufficient to cause abdominal pain
Cause: Narrowing of at least 2 of the 3 visceral branches of the
         aorta (coeliac axis, superior mesenteric or inferior
         mesenteric)

Classical features
  1. Severe upper abdominal colicky pain soon after eating, often
     with borborygmi
  2. Weight loss due to 'food fear'
  3. Initial constipation, progressing to malabsorption
  4. Epigastric bruit conducted to right iliac fossa

CAUSES OF DIARRHOEA

ACUTE

1. **Dietary indiscretion,** e.g. unripe fruit

2. **Drugs (including laxatives)**

3. **Food poisoning**
   Animal
   Plant
   Bacterial (endotoxin or exotoxin)
   Chemical

4. **Gastrointestinal infection**
   Viral, e.g. Rota, Echo
   Bacterial, e.g. *Salmonella, Campylobacter*
   Protozoal, e.g. *Giardia, Amoeba*
   Helminthic, e.g. Tapeworm (esp. *H. nana*)

5. **Allergy** (e.g. to shell-fish)

6. **Psychogenic** (esp. anxiety)

CHRONIC

1. **Irritable bowel syndrome**

2. **Gastric**
   Gastrectomy
   Vagotomy

Linitis plastica
Pernicious anaemia

3. **Intestinal**
   Ulcerative colitis
   Crohn's disease
   Diverticular disease
   Neoplasm, etc.

4. **Malabsorption (q.v.)**

5. **Metabolic**
   Bile-salt diarrhoea (postcholecystectomy)
   Thyrotoxicosis
   Medullary carcinoma of thyroid
   Pellagra
   Gut endocrine tumours (q.v.)

6. **Drugs**
   e.g. purgatives, metformin, etc.

7. ***Clostridium difficile***
   esp. after antibiotics (clindamycin)

8. **Autonomic neuropathy**
   e.g. diabetes (often nocturnal)

9. **Spurious diarrhoea**
   (due to faecal impaction)

GUT ENDOCRINE TUMOURS THAT PRESENT WITH DIARRHOEA

1. * VIP-oma (Werner Morrison syndrome, with hypokalaemia and achlorhydria)
2. Gastrinoma (Zollinger–Ellison syndrome, with intractable peptic ulcers and high gastric acid)
3. Carcinoid tumour (with flush, asthma, R-sided heart lesions and pellagra)
4. Glucagonoma (with necrolytic migratory erythema, diabetes, weight loss, anaemia and stomatitis)
5. Somatostatinoma (with flush, diabetes and hypochlorhydria)

* VIP = vasoactive intestinal peptide

CAUSES OF MALABSORPTION

1. **Inadequate digestion**
   Gastric or intestinal resection
   Bile salt deficiency
   Pancreatic insufficiency (especially fibrocystic disease)

Disorders of enterocyte brush border
  (i) Disaccharidase deficiency
  (ii) Enterokinase deficiency

2. **Parasites**
   Tapeworms
   Giardiasis, *Strongyloides stercoralis*, *Diphyllobothrium latum*

3. **Change in intestinal bacterial flora**

4. **Intestinal hurry or fistulae**

5. **Enterocyte damage**
   Coeliac disease (gluten intolerance)
   Cow's milk intolerance
   Soya flour intolerance
   AIDS (see pp. 59, 215)
   Tropical sprue

6. **Infiltrative disorders**
   Crohn's disease
   Whipple's disease
   Lymphoma or leukaemia
   TB
   Systemic sclerosis
   Systemic mastocytosis
   Alpha-chain disease
   Amyloidosis

7. **Metabolic abnormality**
   Hartnup disease (malabsorption of neutral amino acids)
   Cystinuria (malabsorption of dibasic amino acids)
   Abetalipoproteinaemia
   Carcinoid
   Carcinomatous enteropathy
   Dermatogenic enteropathy (extensive eczema or psoriasis)

8. **Endocrine**
   Addison's hypoadrenalism
   Hypoparathyroidism
   Hyperthyroidism
   Medullary carcinoma of thyroid
   Zollinger–Ellison syndrome
   Werner–Morrison syndrome
   Somatostatinoma
   Diabetes mellitus

9. **Vascular**
   Mesenteric arterial insufficiency
   Chronic venous congestion
   Lymphangiectasia

10. **Drugs**
    Liquid paraffin
    Neomycin, colchicine, cholestyramine, etc.

11. **Radiation enteritis**

CAUSES OF ABNORMAL GUT FLORA ('Stagnant bowel' syndrome)

1. **Abnormalities of gastric function**
    (i) Polya partial gastrectomy—afferent loop syndrome
    (ii) Malfunctioning gastrojejunostomy
    (iii) Pernicious anaemia

2. **Stasis**
    (i) Surgical blind loops
    (ii) Strictures
    (iii) Adhesions
    (iv) Small intestinal diverticulosis
    (v) Abnormal motility
        Systemic sclerosis
        Autonomic neuropathy
        Vagotomy
        Ganglion blocking agents
    (vi) Partial biliary obstruction with cholangitis

3. **Free communications between large and small bowel**
    (i) Gastrocolic fistula
    (ii) Enterocolic fistula
    (iii) Massive intestinal resection

URINARY B_{12}

Urinary B_{12} excretion in the Schilling test

Oral preparation	Pernicious anaemia	Bacterial overgrowth	Ileal disease
B_{12}	Low	Low	Low
B_{12} + intrinsic factor	Normal	Low	Low
B_{12} after antibiotic therapy	Low	Normal	Low

CAUSES OF CALCIFICATION ON ABDOMINAL X-RAY

1. Phleboliths
2. Calcified lymph nodes
3. Calculi (renal, gall-bladder, prostatic)
4. Calcified pancreas, adrenal, liver, kidney, aorta, psoas muscle, costal cartilage, etc.
5. Calcified tumour—dermoid, fibroid, etc.
6. Calcification in abdominal wall, e.g. cysticerci
7. Faecolith
8. Fetus

CAUSE OF A MASS IN R ILIAC FOSSA

1. Appendix abscess
2. Carcinoma caecum
3. Crohn's disease
4. Ileocaecal TB
5. Intussusception
6. Ovarian tumour, tubal pregnancy, etc.
7. Ectopic kidney (might be a transplant)
8. Actinomycosis
9. Carcinoid
10. Amoebiasis
11. Schistosomiasis

COMPLICATIONS AND ASSOCIATIONS OF ULCERATIVE COLITIS

1. **Nutritional deficiencies**
   Anaemia
   Vitamin deficiency
   Dehydration
   Hypokalaemia
   Hypoproteinaemia

2. **Colonic**
   Carcinoma
   Acute toxic dilatation
   Perforation
   Massive bleeding
   Confluent crypt abscesses
   Stricture (in 10%, but rarely causes symptoms)

3. **Anal**
   Haemorrhoids
   Anal fissure
   Anal fistula
   Perianal abscess

4. **Ectodermal**
   Aphthous ulcers
   Clubbing
   Erythema nodosum
   Atopic eczema
   Erythema multiforme
   Pyoderma gangrenosum
   Psoriasis

5. **Arthritis**
   Polyarthritis
   Sacroiliitis
   Ankylosing spondylitis

6. **Ocular**
   Uveitis
   Episcleritis
   Keratitis
   Retinitis
   Retrobulbar neuritis

7. **Hepatic**
   Primary sclerosing cholangitis
   (i) Large duct
   (ii) Small duct
   Cholangiocarcinoma
   Fatty infiltration
   Granulomata
   Abscess (portal bacteraemia)

8. **Pulmonary fibrosis**
   Asthma

9. **Renal**
   Pyelonephritis
   Calculi

10. **Haematological**
    Autoimmune haemolytic
    anaemia
    Iron deficiency

11. **Thrombo-embolism**

12. **Iatrogenic**
    (drugs, transfusions,
    surgery, etc.)

13. **Coeliac disease**

COMPLICATIONS OF CROHN'S DISEASE

1. **Intestinal**
   Small bowel obstruction
   Fistulae, esp. into bladder or vagina
   Perforation
   Suppuration and abscess formation
   Stricture
   Bleeding (usually slow, but may be massive)

2. **Ectodermal**
   Aphthous ulcers
   Clubbing
   Erythema nodosum
   Erythema multiforme
   Pyoderma gangrenosum
   Crohn's disease of mouth or skin (perianal or peri-ileostomy)
   Ectopic Crohn's of skin not contiguous to intestinal mucosa

3. **Nutritional deficiencies** (as for UC, p. 54)
   Due to
   (i)   Decreased food intake
   (ii) Malabsorption—reduction in absorptive surface
                        disaccharidase deficiency
                        altered intestinal flora or intestinal hurry
   (iii) Loss of blood or protein into bowel
   (iv) Increased metabolic requirement

4. **Arthritis**
5. **Ocular** } as for UC (p. 55)
6. **Renal**

7. **Amyloidosis** is commoner in Crohn's than in UC

8. **Hepatic complications** are less common in Crohn's than in UC, but cholesterol gallstones occur

9. **Reduced fertility**

COMPLICATIONS OF PARENTERAL NUTRITION

1. **Complications of central-vein catheterization**
   (i)   Perforation of heart or blood vessel
   (ii)   Thrombosis of vessel
   (iii) Air embolism
   (iv)   Pneumothorax
   (v)   Febrile reactions to pyrogens in tubing
   (vi)   Infections, especially yeast or fungal (and endocarditis)
   (vii) Damage to thoracic duct or brachial plexus

2. **Reactions to nutrients or lack of nutrients**
   (i)   Allergic reaction
   (ii)   Hyperosmolar syndrome with dehydration
   (iii) Hypoglycaemia on rapid cessation of glucose infusion
   (iv)   Hyperchloraemic or lactic acidosis
   (v)   Hypophosphataemia
   (vi)   Fluid overload and electrolyte imbalance
   (vii) Deficiency states
   (viii) Acne conglobata

3. **Cholestatic jaundice**

CAUSES OF HYPOALBUMINAEMIA

1. **Underproduction by the liver**
   (i)   Lack of aminoacid substrate
         a. Maldigestion of dietary protein (e.g. pancreatic
            insufficiency)

    b. Malabsorption
    c. Bacterial overgrowth causing degradation of dietary
       aminoacids
  (ii) Hepatic failure

2. **Haemodilution** (e.g. expanded extracellular fluid in cirrhosis)
3. **Redistribution**
   (i) Into peritoneal cavity (ascites)
  (ii) Into interstitial fluid (increased capillary permeability, e.g.
      in erythroderma)

4. **Loss**
   (i) In urine (nephrotic syndrome)
  (ii) Into the gut (protein-losing enteropathy)
 (iii) From skin surface (burns)

CAUSES OF ASCITES

1. Neoplasm, especially ovarian or alimentary
2. Portal hypertension
3. Hypoalbuminaemia (severe as in nephrotic syndrome)
4. Inferior vena cava or hepatic vein obstruction (Budd–Chiari)
5. Congestive cardiac failure, or constrictive pericarditis
6. Peritonitis
   (i) TB
  (ii) Following perforation (late stage)
 (iii) 'Spontaneous' in cirrhosis
 (iv) Pneumococcal, esp. in young girls
7. Chylous ascites
8. Pancreatitis
9. Haemodialysis or peritoneal dialysis
10. Myxoedema
11. Malnutrition (common in underprivileged countries)
12. Biliary leak (post-surgical)
13. Peritoneal mesothelioma

CAUSES OF PROTEIN-LOSING GASTROENTEROPATHY

1. Giant gastric rugae (Ménétrier's)
2. Ulcerative colitis, Crohn's disease
3. Sprue or coeliac disease
4. Intestinal lipodystrophy (Whipple's)
5. Malignancy, esp. gastric Ca.
6. Intestinal lymphangiectasia or lymphoma
7. Constrictive pericarditis, congestive cardiac failure
8. Hypogammaglobulinaemia
9. Erythroderma

10. 'Allergic gastroenteropathy' (? milk allergy)
11. Villous adenoma of colon

CAUSES OF CONSTIPATION

ACUTE

1. *Ileus*
2. *Obstruction*
3. *'Simple' constipation* due to acute illness, hospital admission, travel, dehydration, low food intake, etc.
4. *Painful anorectal disease,* e.g. fissure

CHRONIC

1. **Disordered intestinal motility**
     (i) *Small faecal residue*, e.g. low fibre diet, dehydration
    (ii) *Over-use of purgatives*
   (iii) *Idiopathic bowel disorder*
           Irritable bowel syndrome (spastic colon)
           Idiopathic slow transit
           Idiopathic megabowel
    (iv) *Secondary to inflammatory bowel disease*
           e.g. diverticulitis, ulcerative colitis
     (v) *Metabolic*
           Early pregnancy
           Hypothyroidism
           Hypercalcaemia
           Hypokalaemia
           Acute intermittent porphyria
           Lead poisoning
    (vi) *Drugs*
           Opiate derivatives
           Ganglion-blockers
           Anticholinergics
           Aluminium hydroxide
           Cholestyramine
           Iron salts
   (vii) *Neuromuscular disease*
           Spinal cord lesions
           Parkinson's disease
           Autonomic neuropathy
           Chagas' disease (toxic destruction of myenteric neurones)
           Systemic sclerosis (gut muscle degeneration)
           Hirschsprung's disease (genetic aganglionosis)

(viii) *Psychiatric*
Depression, psychosis, anorexia nervosa, mental subnormality

2. **Obstruction**
Stricture, tumour, etc.

3. **Rectal dyschezia** (habitual neglect of call to stool)

GAY BOWEL SYNDROME (Infections associated with anal intercourse)

1. **Viruses**
   (i) HIV
   (ii) Human papilloma virus (warts)
   (iii) Herpes simplex
   (iv) Cytomegalovirus
   (v) Epstein–Barr
   (vi) Hepatitis A and B
   (vii) Kaposi's sarcoma (? retrovirus)

2. **Bacteria**
   (i) *Neisseria gonorrhoeae*
   (ii) *Treponema pallidum*
   (iii) *Chlamydia trachomatis* (proctitis)
   (iv) Enteric infections (Shigella, Salmonella, Campylobacter)

3. **Protozoa**
   (i) *Giardia lamblia*
   (ii) *Entamoeba histolytica*

4. **Helminths**
   e.g. *Enterobius vermicularis*

5. **Arthropods**
   (i) *Sarcoptes scabiei* (scabies)
   (ii) *Phthirus pubis* (crab-lice)

GASTROINTESTINAL MANIFESTATIONS OF AIDS

1. **Infections**
   As above, *plus*:

Opportunistic infections
   (i) Candida (oral or oesophageal), herpes simplex, CMV, etc.
   (ii) Cryptosporidiosis (opportunistic coccidian protozoa, causing weight loss and severe watery diarrhoea)

(iii)   *Toxoplasma gondii* and *Isospora belli*
(iv)   *Mycobacterium avium intracellulare* (liver or bowel)
(v)   Oral hairy leukoplakia

2. **Kaposi's sarcoma**
    May involve pharynx, oesophagus, stomach, duodenum or colon

3. **Lymphoma** (B cell)
    May involve CNS, marrow or gut

4. **Partial villous atrophy**
    With malabsorption despite no identifiable pathogen
    Cachexia is a major feature in Africa

5. **Liver and biliary system**
    Viral hepatitis concurrent infection
    Mycobacterium avium intracellulare
    Sclerosing cholangitis

CAUSES OF HEPATOMEGALY

1. **Raised venous pressure**
    Congestive cardiac failure
    Constrictive pericarditis
    Tricuspid stenosis
    Hepatic vein obstruction (Budd–Chiari)

2. **Degenerative**
    Fatty infiltration and early cirrhosis (esp. alcoholic)
    Reye's syndrome

3. **Myeloproliferative disease**

4. **Neoplastic**
    Primary (hepatoma, etc.)
    Metastases
    Lymphoma

5. **Infective**
    Viral—Infective and serum hepatitis
          Infectious mononucleosis
    Bacterial—Hepatic abscess
              TB, syphilis
              Brucellosis
              Weil's disease

Protozoal—Amoebic abscess
          Malaria
          Toxoplasmosis
          Kala-azar
Parasitic—Hydatid cyst

6. **Storage disorders**
   Amyloidosis
   Wilson's disease
   Gaucher's
   Niemann–Pick's
   Histiocytosis X (Langerhans cell)
   Glycogen storage disease
   Haemochromatosis
   Hurler's (gargoylism)

7. **Biliary obstruction**

8. **Sarcoidosis**

9. **Rheumatoid disease**

10. **Congenital**
    Polycystic disease
    Congenital hepatic fibrosis

11. **Apparent**
    Riedel's lobe (palpable but not hepatomegaly)
    Hyperinflation of lungs

Causes of a hard knobbly liver
1. Carcinoma metastases
2. Cirrhosis with hepatoma
3. Polycystic liver
4. Hydatid cysts
5. Hepar lobatum (syphilis)

Causes of hepatosplenomegaly
1. Infective, e.g. infectious mononucleosis
2. Myeloproliferative, e.g. myelofibrosis, chronic myeloid leukaemia
3. Some causes of portal hypertension, e.g. Budd–Chiari syndrome
4. Reticuloses
5. Storage diseases, e.g. Gaucher's disease, amyloidosis
6. Anaemia, e.g. PA, sickle-cell anaemia in children

Causes of acute liver failure
1. Viral hepatitis (A, B, E and ? C)
2. Toxins, e.g. carbon tetrachloride, *Amanita phalloides*
3. Drugs, e.g. paracetamol overdose, aspirin (Reye's syndrome)

4. Anaesthetics, e.g. halothane
5. Metabolic, e.g. Wilson's disease
6. Acute fatty liver of pregnancy

CAUSES OF JAUNDICE WITH URAEMIA

1. *Infections*
   (i)   Gram-negative septicaemia
   (ii) Leptospirosis icterohaemorrhagiae (Weil's)
   (iii) Yellow fever
2. *Drugs and toxins*
   (i)   Direct toxicity, e.g. carbon tetrachloride, paracetamol
   (ii) Hypersensitivity, e.g. penicillin
3. *Hepatorenal syndrome*
   Oliguria secondary to hepatic failure, usually following biliary tract surgery or cirrhosis
4. Haemolytic-uraemic syndrome
5. Incompatible blood transfusion
6. Toxaemia of pregnancy
7. Other causes of 'shock' (p. 15)

CIRRHOSIS

Cirrhosis is characterized by hepatic parenchymal damage with fibrosis and nodular regeneration throughout the liver, accompanied by distortion of the normal lobular pattern

CAUSES

1. **Infection**
   (i)   Viral hepatitis B and C
   (ii) ? Other viruses
   (iii) Schistosomiasis
   (iv) Congenital syphilis

2. **Toxins**
   (i)   Alcohol
   (ii) Drugs, e.g. methotrexate

3. **Prolonged cholestasis**
   e.g. biliary stricture

4. **Immunological**
   (i)   Primary biliary (Hanot's)
   (ii) Autoimmune hepatitis
   (iii) Primary sclerosing cholangitis

5. Metabolic
  (i) Haemochromatosis
  (ii) Hepatolenticular degeneration (Wilson's)
  (iii) Galactosaemia
  (iv) Fructosaemia
  (v) Glycogen storage disease
  (vi) Tyrosinosis
  (vii) α_1-Antitrypsin deficiency

6. Venous stasis
  (i) Prolonged congestive cardiac failure
  (ii) Hepatic vein occlusion

7. Miscellaneous
  (i) Cystic fibrosis
  (ii) Secondary biliary cirrhosis
  (iii) Hereditary haemorrhagic telangiectasia (Osler's)
  (iv) Sickle-cell disease
  (v) Jejunoileal bypass (for obesity)
  (vi) Coeliac disease
  (vii) Anorexia nervosa

8. Idiopathic

Complications of chronic biliary obstruction
  1. Liver cell dysfunction
  2. Acute oliguric renal failure (especially in the elderly)
  3. Metabolic bone disease (osteomalacia or osteoporosis) and hyperparathyroidism
  4. Vitamin K deficiency
  5. Hyperlipidaemia
  6. Infection of biliary tree and septicaemia
  7. Pigmentation
  8. Pruritus
  9. Weight loss due to malabsorption

Disorders associated with primary biliary cirrhosis
  1. Systemic sclerosis (including CRST syndrome)
  2. Sjogren's syndrome, rheumatoid disease or SLE
  3. Thyroiditis
  4. Renal tubular acidosis
  5. Lichen planus

Causes of intrahepatic cholestasis

In children
Biliary atresia
Neonatal (giant cell) hepatitis

Galactosaemia
Mucoviscidosis
α_1-Antitrypsin deficiency
Viral hepatitis
Byler disease (a genetic bile duct disorder)

In adults
Drugs (e.g. androgens, oestrogens, phenothiazines)
Viral hepatitis
Primary biliary cirrhosis
Alcohol
Pregnancy
Primary sclerosing cholangitis
Cirrhosis
Idiopathic

PORTAL HYPERTENSION

CAUSES

1. **Extrahepatic presinusoidal (Portal vein thrombosis)**
   Umbilical sepsis, exchange transfusion in neonates
   Suppurative pylephlebitis
   Portal lymphadenopathy (Ca. metastasis, lymphoma, etc.)
   Thrombophilia, e.g. polycythaemia

2. **Intrahepatic presinusoidal**
   Schistosomiasis
   Sarcoid, Hodgkin's, leukaemic infiltrates
   Congenital hepatic fibrosis

3. **Intrahepatic postsinusoidal**
   Cirrhosis
   Veno-occlusive disease (Jamaican bush-tea)

4. **Extrahepatic postsinusoidal**
   Hepatic vein obstruction (Budd–Chiari)
   Inferior vena caval occlusion
   Constrictive pericarditis
When obstruction is presinusoidal, hepatic function is relatively
unimpaired, and bleeding from varices does not cause liver failure

HEPATIC ENCEPHALOPATHY

Cerebral dysfunction which can complicate all forms of liver disease
and which particularly affects consciousness. The mean EEG
frequency is slowed, nitrogenous substances are retained in the
brain and giant astrocytes proliferate

Clinical types of hepatic encephalopathy
1. *Chronic portasystemic encephalopathy*
2. *Cirrhosis with a precipitant*
   e.g. Diuresis
         Haemorrhage
         Paracentesis abdominis
         Diarrhoea and vomiting
         Surgery
         Alcohol
         Sedatives (esp. opiates and benzodiazepine)
         Infections (esp. infected ascites)
3. *Acute liver failure*

Factors affecting hepatic encephalopathy
1. Portasystemic collaterals
   (i) Extrahepatic, e.g. varices, shunt
   (ii) Intrahepatic, e.g. around cirrhotic nodules or transjugular intrahepatic percutaneous shunting (TIPS)
2. Nitrogenous content of intestines
3. Bacterial action on colonic contents
4. Liver cell function

PATTERNS OF HEPATOCYTE INJURY

1. **Direct**
   Characterized by mitochondrial damage, central necrosis and, usually, fatty change
   (i) Alcohol
       Obesity   } Predominantly mitochondrial
       Diabetes mellitus   damage
       Wilson's disease
   (ii) Reye's syndrome
       Tetracycline toxicity   } Damage to mitochondria and
       Fatty liver of pregnancy   ribosomes
       Cytotoxic drugs
   (iii) Metabolite-related, e.g. isoniazid is converted to an acylating agent
   (iv) Anoxia, e.g. 'shock' or hepatic venous obstruction
   (v) Heavy-metal escape from lysosomes, e.g. haemochromatosis

2. **Immunological**
   Characterized by damage to cell membranes, piecemeal necrosis of periportal hepatocytes and mononuclear infiltrates
   (i) Chronic active hepatitis
   (ii) Primary biliary cirrhosis
   (iii) Drug reactions, e.g. halothane

3. **Cholestatic**
   Characterized by retention of bile in liver cells and canaliculi, with secondary effects on other organelles
   (i)   Extrahepatic, e.g. due to stones in bile duct
   (ii) Intrahepatic, e.g. due to sex hormones

HEPATITIS

Viral causes
1. *Hepatitis A:* an enterovirus in the picorna group spread by the faecal–oral route
2. *Hepatitis B:* DNA virus, highly infective by the blood-borne route, unique in the human
3. *Hepatitis C:* RNA virus related to flavi and toga viruses. Accounts for 90% of post-transfusion hepatitis and around 50% of sporadic non-A, non-B. Common among intravenous drug users
4. *Hepatitis D:* requires co-infection with hepatitis B (provision of the HBsAg coat)
5. *Hepatitis E:* Enterovirus, can cause epidemics. Found worldwide, causes fulminant hepatitis especially amongst pregnant women (mortality ~20%)
6. *Hepatitis F:* Sporadic cause of fulminant hepatitis. Existence not fully established
7. *Hepatitis G:* giant cell hepatitis seen in children
   ? paramyxovirus
8. *Other viruses* such as EBV, CMV, measles

Chronic sequelae of viral hepatitis
1. Chronic persistent hepatitis/chronic active hepatitis
2. Autoimmune hepatitis (q.v.)
3. Asymptomatic carrier state
4. Cirrhosis
5. Primary liver cancer (after hepatitis B and C)

AUTOIMMUNE HEPATITIS (formerly called autoimmune chronic active hepatitis)

A chronic disease, predominantly affecting the liver, with continuing damage to hepatocytes and with evidence of abnormal immunological activity

Possible aetiological factors
1. Viral hepatitis
2. Drugs—Oxyphenisatin, methyldopa, isoniazid
3. Other chronic liver disease, especially alcoholic
4. α_1-Antitrypsin deficiency

CLASSIFICATION OF AUTOIMMUNE HEPATITIS

Disease	AMA	ANA	LKM	SLA	SMA	ANCA
PBC	100%	Common	—	—	Rare	Occas.
CAH Classical (subgroup I)	Occas.	100%	—	—	Common	Occas.
CAH LKM (subgroup II)	—	Rare	100%	—	Rare	—
CAH SLA (subgroup III)	Occas.	Rare	—	100%	Occas.	—
PSC	—	Occas.	—	—	Occas.	80%

AMA Antimitochondrial antibody, ANA Antinuclear antibody, LKM Liver, kidney, microsomal, SLA Soluble liver antigen, SMA Smooth muscle antibody, ANCA Antineutrophilic cytoplasmic antibody, PBC Primary biliary cirrhosis, CAH Chronic active hepatitis, PSC Primary sclerosing cholangitis

LIVER TUMOURS

CAUSES OF PRIMARY LIVER TUMOURS

Hepatocellular Ca.
1. Cirrhosis
2. Toxins
    (i) Aflatoxin (a metabolite of a mould which grows on rice and peanuts)
    (ii) Nitrosamines
3. Anabolic androgens
4. Viral hepatitis (B and C)

Cholangiocarcinoma
1. Primary sclerosing cholangitis
2. Parasitic infestation of biliary tree
    (i) Liver fluke—*Clonorchis sinensis*
    (ii) Schistosomiasis

Angiosarcoma
1. Previous 'Thorotrast' injection (for radiography)
2. Arsenic
3. Vinyl chloride monomer

ALPHA-FETOPROTEIN (AFP)

Occurs in plasma in:
1. Normal fetus
2. Elevated maternal AFP may indicate fetal neural-tube defect, twin pregnancy, intrauterine death, threatened abortion or subsequent low birth-weight

3. Hepatoma (in 90%)
4. Infective hepatitis, cirrhosis or liver metastases
5. Occasionally in primary Ca. of stomach, ovary or testis

SOME 'METABOLIC' EFFECTS OF LIVER CELL CARCINOMA
1. Hypoglycaemia
2. Hypercalcaemia
3. Hyperlipidaemia
4. Hypertrophic pulmonary osteoarthropathy
5. Erythrocytosis
6. Dysfibrinogenaemia
7. Porphyria cutanea tarda
8. Carcinoid syndrome
9. Sexual precocity

HAEMOCHROMATOSIS

Haemosiderosis implies a pathological increase in tissue iron levels, but is not necessarily accompanied by cell damage

Haemochromatosis implies increased tissue iron with accompanying cell damage

Causes of haemochromatosis
1. *Primary* (dominant with incomplete penetrance)
2. *Secondary*
   (i)   Multiple blood transfusions
   (ii) Inability to utilize iron
         a. Sideroblastic anaemia
         b. Thalassaemia
         c. Sickle-cell anaemia
   (iii) Increased iron ingestion (e.g. Kaffir beer made in iron cooking pots)
   (iv) Liver disease, especially due to alcohol
   (v)   Porta-caval shunt
   (vi) Porphyria cutanea tarda
   (vii) Xanthinuria
   (viii) Congenital transferrin deficiency

LIVER DISEASE DUE TO DRUGS OR CHEMICALS

1. *Hepatic necrosis due to toxins*
   Halogenated hydrocarbons
   Heavy metals
   Iron or paracetamol overdose

2. *Hepatitis*
   Monoamine oxidase inhibitors
   Antidepressants (e.g. lofepramine)
   Antirheumatic drugs
   Anticonvulsants
3. *Cholestasis*
   (i) Hypersensitivity, e.g. chlorpromazine
   (ii) Steroid-cholestasis, e.g. 17-methyltestosterone
   (iii) Flucloxacillin
4. *Generalized hypersensitivity,* e.g. antibiotics
5. *Hepatic vein occlusion*
   Plant toxins ('bush teas')
   Oral contraceptives
6. *Fibrosis or cirrhosis*
   Cytotoxins, especially methotrexate
7. *Interference with normal bilirubin pathway* (normal liver histology)
   (i) Haemolysis, e.g. methyldopa
   (ii) Decreased uptake, e.g. filix mas
   (iii) Conjugation defect, e.g. novobiocin
   (iv) Competition with bilirubin, e.g. X-ray contrast media
   (v) Protein-binding release, e.g. salicylates
8. *Hepatic hyperplasia, adenoma or carcinoma*
   Anabolic and androgenic steroids
   Oral contraceptives
   Nitrosamines
9. *Fibrosis or angiosarcoma*
   Arsenic
   Thorotrast
   Vinyl chloride
10. *Secondary sclerosing cholangitis*
    Fluorodeoxyuridine

FAMILIAL NON-HAEMOLYTIC JAUNDICE

Unconjugated
1. *Gilbert's*
   Decreased uptake of bilirubin by liver cell
   Mild intermittent jaundice
2. *Primary 'shunt' hyperbilirubinaemia*
   Increased production of bilirubin in marrow
   Very rare
3. *Crigler–Najjar*
   Hepatic glucuronyl-transferase deficiency
   Poor prognosis. Extremely rare
4. *Familial neonatal hyperbilirubinaemia*
   Glucuronyl-transferase inhibitor in serum

5. *Breast milk jaundice*
   Glucuronyl-transferase inhibitor in breast milk

Conjugated
 1. *Dubin–Johnson*
    Mild intermittent jaundice
    Brown pigment in liver cells
    Characteristic BSP test with secondary rise at 2 hr due to
    re-entry of conjugated bilirubin into blood
 2. *Rotor*
    Similar but without hepatic pigmentation
 3. *Summerskill and Walshe*
    Recurrent cholestasis of unknown cause

PANCREATITIS

CAUSES OF ACUTE PANCREATITIS

 1. Biliary tract disease, including gallstones
 2. Alcohol
 3. Idiopathic
 4. Metabolic
     (i) Hyperparathyroidism
     (ii) Hypercalcaemia
     (iii) Hyperlipidaemia
     (iv) Pregnancy and postpartum
 5. Trauma, ERCP or biliary surgery
 6. Congenital defects
    e.g. obstructed pancreatic duct
 7. Drugs
     (i) Morphine
     (ii) Steroids
     (iii) Thiazide diuretics or frusemide
     (iv) Azathioprine
     (v) Sulphonamides
     (vi) Oestrogens
     (vii) Tetracyclines
 8. Viral
     (i) Mumps
     (ii) Infectious hepatitis
     (iii) Infectious mononucleosis
 9. Parasitic
     (i) *Ascaris lumbricoides*
     (ii) *Clonorchis sinensis*
10. Vascular disease
11. Carcinoma of pancreas
12. Hypothermia

CAUSES OF CHRONIC PANCREATITIS

1. Alcoholism
2. Malnutrition
3. Cystic fibrosis
4. Familial (sometimes with cyclical neutropenia)
5. Idiopathic

INDICATIONS FOR ORTHOTOPIC LIVER TRANSPLANTATION

1. **Autoimmune**
   Primary biliary cirrhosis
   Primary sclerosing cholangitis
   Autoimmune hepatitis

2. **Acute/subacute hepatic failure**
   Viral
   Drugs, e.g. paracetamol
   Metabolic liver disease, e.g. Wilson's

3. **Chronic hepatitis**
   Hepatitis B and C
   Drug-induced
   Cryptogenic

4. **Alcohol**
   Acute alcoholic hepatitis
   Cirrhosis

5. **Inborn errors of metabolism**
   α_1-Antitrypsin deficiency
   Haemochromatosis
   Gaucher's disease
   Haemophilia
   Cystic fibrosis, etc. (many others)

6. **Others**
   Biliary atresia (commonest paediatric indication)
   Budd–Chiari syndrome
   Neoplasia (poor long term survival)

Haematology

NORMAL VALUES IN HAEMATOLOGY

See note on SI units on page 237
Imperial units are given in parentheses

Haemoglobin
Men   13.0–18.0 g/dl (g.%)
Women   11.5–16.5 g/dl (g.%)

Red cell count (RBC)
Men   4.5–6.5 x 10^{12}/l (4.5–6.5 million/c.mm)
Women   3.9–5.6 x 10^{12}/l (3.9–5.6 million/c.mm)

Haematocrit (PCV)
Men   0.40–0.54
Women   0.36–0.47
(Calculated as RBC x MCV ÷ 1000)

Mean cell volume (MCV)
Adults 80–98 fl (cμ)

Mean cell haemoglobin (MCH)
Adults 27–32 pg
(Calculated as Hb x 10 ÷ RBC)

Mean corpuscular haemoglobin concentration (MCHC)
Adults 31–35 g/dl (g.%)
(Calculated as Hb ÷ PCV)

Leukocytes
Adults 4–10 x 10^9/l (4000–10 000/c.mm)
Differential: Neutrophils 2500–7500 x 10^6/l
                Lymphocytes 1500–3500 x 10^6/l
                Monocytes 200–800 x 10^6/l
                Eosinophils 40–440 x 10^6/l
                Basophils 0–100 x 10^6/l

Platelets
150–400 x 10^9/l (150 000–400 000/c.mm)

Reticulocytes
0.2–2%

Plasma viscosity
1.50–1.72 cp
Parallels ESR but is unaffected by age, sex or anaemia

ESR (Westergren)
Men–up to 5 mm/h
Women–up to 7 mm/h

RED CELL SHAPE

Cell types	Causes
1. Echinocyte ('Burr' cell)	1. Uraemia 2. Ca. stomach or bleeding peptic ulcer 3. Post transfusion with old blood 4. Low-potassium red cells 5. Pyruvate kinase deficiency
2. Stomatocyte ('Mouth' cell)	1. Hereditary stomatocytosis 2. Liver disease 3. RBC sodium-pump defect
3. Codocyte ('Target' cell) 'Target' on dried film Bell-shaped on scanning electron microscopy	1. Obstructive liver disease 2. Haemoglobinopathies 3. Thalassaemia 4. Iron deficiency 5. Post-splenectomy 6. LCAT deficiency
4. Acanthocyte ('Spur' cell)	1. Abetalipoproteinaemia 2. Alcoholic liver disease 3. Post-splenectomy 4. Malabsorption

Cell types	Causes
5. **Spherocyte** ('Spherical' cell)	1. Hereditary spherocytosis 2. Immune haemolytic anaemia 3. Heinz body haemolytic anaemia 4. Post-transfusion 5. Water-dilution anaemia 6. Fragmentation haemolysis
6. **Elliptocyte** ('Oval' cell)	1. Hereditary elliptocytosis 2. Thalassaemia 3. Iron deficiency 4. Myelophthistic anaemia 5. Megaloblastic anaemia
7. **Schizocyte** ('Helmet' cell) 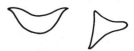	1. Microangiopathic haemolytic anaemia 2. Heart valve haemolysis (e.g. prosthesis) 3. Severe burns or calcification 4. March haemoglobinuria
8. **Drepanocyte** ('Sickle' cell) Varying spiculated shapes e.g. 'Sickle' or 'Holly-leaf'	Haemoglobinopathies: SS, S-trait, SC, etc. 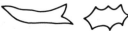
9. **Dacrocyte** ('Teardrop' cell)	1. Myelofibrosis with myeloid metaplasia 2. Myelophthistic anaemia 3. Thalassaemia
10. **Leptocyte** ('Wafer' cell)	1. Thalassaemia 2. Obstructive liver disease

NB Myelophthistic anaemia is due to a disrupted vascular pattern of the marrow. Causes include metastasis, lymphoma, myelofibrosis and TB

RBC abnormalities produced by absent spleen
1. Target cells
2. Acanthocytes
3. Schizocytes
4. Howell–Jolly bodies

RED CELL INCLUSION BODIES

Howell–Jolly bodies
Nuclear remnants seen as small dense purple particles at the periphery

Causes
1. Splenectomy and splenic atrophy (p. 88)
2. Dyshaemopoietic states: leukaemia, megaloblastic anaemia, etc.

Pappenheimer bodies
Fe-containing granules in siderocytes

Causes
1. Sideroblastic anaemia (q.v.)
2. Haemolytic anaemia, esp. after splenectomy

Heinz bodies
Occur in reticulocyte preparations as peripheral, rounded, dark blue bodies (globin denatured by oxidants)

Causes
1. Haemolytic anaemia due to oxidant drugs and chemicals
2. RBC enzyme defects, e.g. G6PD deficiency
3. Rare haemoglobinopathies ('unstable haemoglobins', e.g. Hb Koln) after splenectomy

Causes of methaemoglobinaemia
1. *Genetic*
   NADH-Diaphorase deficiency
   Abnormal α or β chain

2. *Acquired*
   Phenacetin
   Sulphonamides (including dapsone)
   Primaquine
   Sulphasalazine
   Shoe polish
   Aniline dyes

HYPOCHROMIC ANAEMIA

Causes of hypochromic anaemia other than Fe deficiency
1. Infection
2. Rh. arthritis ⎫ though more often normochromic
3. Uraemia ⎬
4. Malignancy ⎭
5. Thalassaemia major and minor
6. Sideroblastic anaemia (q.v.)

Causes of sideroblastic anaemia
(Defined as hypochromic anaemia with 'ring sideroblasts' in the marrow)
1. *Hereditary*
   Usually sex-linked. May or may not respond to pyridoxine
2. *Idiopathic*
3. *Drugs*
   (i) Alcohol
   (ii) Antituberculous drugs
   (iii) Chloramphenicol
4. *Lead poisoning*
5. *Myeloproliferative disease*
6. *Haemolytic anaemia*
7. *Miscellaneous non-haematological disorders*
   (i) Malabsorption
   (ii) Infections
   (iii) Collagen-vascular disease
   (iv) Carcinoma
   (v) Cutaneous porphyria

Haematological effects of lead poisoning
1. Anaemia
2. Basophilic stippling
3. Reticulocytosis
4. Erythroid hyperplasia and 'ring sideroblasts' in marrow
5. Increased Se Fe in adults
6. 'Fast' Hb (on electrophoresis) in children with Fe deficiency

HAEMOLYTIC ANAEMIAS

CLASSIFICATION

Hereditary
1. *Erythrocyte membrane defect*
   Hereditary spherocytosis, elliptocytosis or stomatocytosis
2. *Erythrocyte metabolism defect*
   (i) Embden—Meyerhof pathway, e.g. pyruvate kinase deficiency
   (ii) Hexose-monophosphate shunt defect, e.g. glucose-6-phosphate dehydrogenase (G6PD), or glutathione deficiency
3. *Abnormal haemoglobins*
   (i) Stable Hb variants, e.g. Hb-S, Hb-C or combinations of Hb-S with thalassaemia
   Sickle cell disease (Hb-S homozygotes) causes severe anaemia, the other forms are milder
   (ii) Unstable Hb variants, e.g. Hb-Koln, Hb-Zurich, Hb-Hammersmith
   These are rare, but can cause severe anaemia even in the heterozygote state

4. *Impaired globin synthesis*
   α or β-thalassaemia (p. 78)
Haemolysis is important in homozygotes, or in heterozygotes who also have an abnormal Hb such as Hb-S or Hb-C

Acquired
1. *Autoimmune* (RBC Antibody, with Coombs test positive)
   (i) Warm antibody
      a. Idiopathic
      b. Methyldopa injection
      c. Secondary to many 'immune' disorders, e.g. SLE, RA, PN or lymphoma
   (ii) Cold antibody
      a. Idiopathic cold-haemagglutinin, especially in the elderly.
      b. Secondary to malignant lymphoma (continuous Ab production) or to infection such as mycoplasma or infectious mononucleosis (transient Ab production). The antibody is IgM
   (iii) Paroxysmal cold haemoglobinuria
      a. Idiopathic; acute transient or chronic
      b. Secondary—acute transient after viral infection (measles, varicella); chronic after syphilis
      The antibody is IgG (the Donath–Landsteiner antibody)
2. *Non-autoimmune*
   (i) Drug-induced
      a. Toxic chemicals:　Arsene, lead, naphthalene
      　　　　　　　　　　　Snake or spider venoms
      　　　　　　　　　　　Plant toxins, e.g. male fern
      b. Overdose of drugs, e.g. phenacetin, dapsone. The erythrocytes are normal
      c. Idiosyncrasy, e.g. antimalarials, sulphonamides or sulphones in G6PD deficiency
      d. Hypersensitivity: Antibodies form against the drug or its metabolites, e.g. in prolonged high dose penicillin therapy this drug is absorbed to the erythrocyte, and drug antibodies then cause haemolysis
   (ii) *Alloimmunity* Passive transfer of alloantibody from one subject to another, e.g. haemolytic disease of newborn, or transfusion of group O blood (with anti-A activity) to group A recipients
   (iii) *Mechanical*
      a. Cardiac open heart surgery, prosthetic valve, etc.
      b. Microangiopathic haemolytic anaemia (q.v.)
      c. 'March' (exertional) haemoglobinuria
   (iv) *Paroxysmal nocturnal haemoglobinuria*
      The basic defect is increased sensitivity to erythrocyte lysis by complement. Confirmed by the acid serum lysis test

(Ham's test). Associated with aplastic anaemia or venous thrombosis in some cases
   (v) *Secondary non-autoimmune haemolytic anaemia*
      A miscellaneous group, in which the mechanism of haemolysis may be obscure
      a. *Infections,* e.g. malaria (esp. Blackwater fever), bartonellosis (Oroya fever) and *Clostridium welchii*
      b. Lymphoma, leukaemia, liver or kidney disease
      c. Hypersplenism
      d. Severe burns or radiation
      e. Secondary to RBC metabolic defect, e.g. megaloblastic anaemia or iron deficiency

Clinical manifestations of G6P Dehydrogenase deficiency
1. Drug-induced haemolysis
2. Infection-induced haemolysis
3. Broad bean-induced haemolysis (Favism)
4. Chronic non-spherocytic haemolysis
5. Neonatal jaundice (especially after Vit. K in Greeks and Chinese)

CAUSES OF MICROANGIOPATHIC HAEMOLYTIC ANAEMIA (MHA)

Haemolysis is due to trauma to circulating red cells which become entangled in fibrin threads in small blood vessels. The red cells are characteristically fragmented and bizarrely shaped
   In some cases the haemolysis is due to disseminated intravascular coagulation
1. Haemolytic uraemia syndrome
   Thrombocytopenia, acute renal failure and MHA (usually in infants)
2. Thrombotic thrombocytopenic purpura (Moschowitz)
3. Septicaemia
4. Acute glomerulonephritis
5. Eclampsia or postpartum
6. Disseminated carcinomatosis

THALASSAEMIA SYNDROMES

A heterogeneous group of hereditary disorders characterized by decreased synthesis of either the α or the β chain of adult HbA ($\alpha_2\beta_2$). There is a wide spectrum of clinical disorders, since α and β thalassaemia and haemoglobinopathies may coexist

Factors in the production of the anaemia
1. The Hb deficit produces a hypochromic microcytic anaemia
2. The relative excess of α or β chains precipitates in the red cell, forming inclusion bodies (Heinz bodies) which damage the RBC membrane and cause haemolysis
3. Folic acid deficiency

4. Mitochondrial iron deposition
5. Hypersplenism

CAUSES OF MEGALOBLASTIC ANAEMIA

A. Folate deficiency
1. *Inadequate diet* (esp. alcoholics and old people)
2. *Malabsorption from upper intestine*
3. *Increased demand*
   - (i) Infancy or pregnancy
   - (ii) Increased cell turnover
       Myeloproliferative disease
       Malignancy or lymphoma
       Chronic haemolysis
       Chronic inflammation, e.g. rheumatoid disease
       Erythroderma
4. *Antifolate drugs*
   - (i) Dihydrofolate reductase inhibitors
       Methotrexate, pyrimethamine, trimethoprim
   - (ii) Impaired absorption
       Cholestyramine, sulphasalazine
   - (iii) Uncertain mechanism
       Anticonvulsants, ethanol, oral contraceptives

B. Vitamin B_{12} deficiency
1. *Malabsorption*
   - (i) Lack of intrinsic factor
       Addisonian PA
       Partial or total gastrectomy
       Gastric atrophy due to gastritis
       Congenital PA with normal mucosa
       Rarely associated with polyendocrinopathy
   - (ii) General malabsorption (p. 51)
   - (iii) Specific B_{12} malabsorption
       Ileal resection
       Ileal TB, Crohn's or ulcerative colitis
       Chelating agents (ingested phytates)
       Rarely congenital, with proteinuria
   - (iv) B_{12} utilization by bacteria or parasites
       Blind-loop syndrome, diverticulosis, etc.
       Diphyllobothrium latum (fish tape-worm)
2. *Inadequate diet*
   Rare except in vegans and starvation
3. *Drugs*
   PAS, colchicine, neomycin, metformin

C. With normal folate and B_{12}
   - (i) Cytotoxic drugs, e.g. hydroxyurea, cytosine arabinoside

(ii)   Hereditary orotic aciduria (responds to uridine)
(iii) Erythroleukaemia

Causes of macrocytic anaemia with normoblastic marrow

1. Haemolysis   ⎫
2. Haemorrhage   ⎬ since reticulocytes are macrocytes
3. Leukaemia   ⎭
4. Aplastic anaemia
5. Marrow infiltration or replacement (see below)
6. Cytotoxic drugs, e.g. azathioprine
7. Sideroblastic anaemia
8. Alcohol ingestion
9. Cirrhosis
10. Myxoedema or hypopituitarism
11. Protein deficiency
12. Scurvy

Causes of reduction in normal marrow activity

1. *Nutritional defect*
   (i)   Fe, B_{12}, folate or pyridoxine deficiency
   (ii) Kwashiorkor
2. *Endocrine defect*
   (i)   Erythropoietin deficiency (renal disease)
   (ii) Hypothyroidism
   (iii) Hypopituitarism
3. *Haemopoietic cell defect*
   (i)   Aplastic anaemia (p. 81)
   (ii) Red-cell aplasia
4. *Marrow infiltration*
   (i)   Myelofibrosis (and osteosclerosis)
   (ii)   Malignant lymphoma
   (iii) Myelomatosis
   (iv)   Metastatic carcinoma
   (v)   Leukaemia
   (vi)   Histiocytosis X (Langerhans cell)
   (vii) Lipidoses (Gaucher's, Niemann–Pick's)
   (viii) Miliary TB

LEUKOPENIA

CAUSES OF NEUTROPENIA ($<2.5 \times 10^9$ neutrophils/l)

1. Pancytopenia (q.v.)
2. Infections
   (i)   Viral
   (ii) Bacterial: typhoid, brucellosis, miliary TB, overwhelming
         septicaemia
   (iii) Rickettsial: typhus
   (iv) Protozoal: malaria, kala-azar

3. Drugs causing selective neutropenia: thiouracil, etc.
4. Megaloblastic anaemia
5. Hypothyroidism, thyrotoxicosis, hypopituitarism
6. Cirrhosis
7. Alcoholism
8. Idiopathic (chronic or periodic)

CAUSES OF PANCYTOPENIA

1. Aplastic anaemia (q.v.)
2. Acute leukaemia (in subleukaemic phase)
3. Marrow infiltration:
   (i) Malignant lymphoma
   (ii) Metastatic carcinoma
   (iii) Myelomatosis
   (iv) Myelosclerosis (in late stages)
4. Hypersplenism
5. Pernicious anaemia
6. SLE
7. Rarely disseminated TB

Types of aplastic anaemia

A. *With thrombocytopenia* (WCC may be low or normal)
   1. Chronic acquired
      (i) Idiopathic
      (ii) Drugs or toxins
          Dose-related, e.g. benzene, cytotoxics
          Idiosyncratic, e.g. chloramphenicol, phenylbutazone,
          mianserin, carbimazole
      (iii) Irradiation
   2. Transient, following infection (especially hepatitis)
   3. Congenital pancytopenia (Fanconi's)
   NB a. Pancytopenic aplastic anaemia may be complicated by
      paroxysmal nocturnal haemoglobinuria or leukaemia
      b. Chloramphenicol may produce either an early dose-related
      reversible marrow depression or, more rarely, an idiosyncratic
      severe aplastic anaemia of late onset

B. *Red cell aplasia* (with normal WCC and platelets)
   1. Chronic acquired
      (i) Idiopathic
      (ii) Immune, with thymoma and myasthenia gravis
   2. Secondary to renal disease
   3. Associated with haemolysis, infection or riboflavin deficiency
   4. Congenital (Diamond–Blackfan)

LEUKOCYTOSIS

Causes of leukocytosis (>10 x 10^9/l in adults)
1. Physiological
    (i) Infancy
    (ii) Pregnancy and postpartum
2. Infection
3. Haemorrhage
4. Trauma, burns, surgery
5. Myeloproliferative disease
6. Malignancy
7. Myocardial infarction and paroxysmal tachycardia
8. Drugs: steroids, digitalis, adrenaline
9. Chemicals: lead, mercury, carbon monoxide
10. 'Collagen-vascular' disease
11. Metabolic disturbances: renal failure, gout, diabetic coma, eclampsia, etc.
12. Miscellaneous: haemolysis, serum sickness, acute anoxia, spider venom, etc.

Causes of myeloid leukaemoid reaction (WCC>50 x 10^9/l or myelocytes or myeloblasts present in peripheral blood)
1. Infections, esp. in children and after splenectomy
2. Leuko-erythroblastic anaemia (q.v.)
3. Malignancy
4. Acute haemolysis

Features of leuko-erythroblastic anaemia
Normocytic, normochromic anaemia with poikilocytes, dacrocytes, reticulocytes and myelocytes seen on peripheral film

Causes of leuko-erythroblastic anaemia
1. Metastases to bone
2. Myelosclerosis
3. Myelomatosis
4. Malignant lymphoma
5. Granulomatous marrow, e.g. TB
6. Gaucher's, Niemann–Pick's, histiocytosis X (Langerhans cell)
7. Severe infections

Causes of lymphocytosis (>3.5 x 10^9/l)
1. Infections
    (i) Viral: infectious mononucleosis; infective hepatitis; infectious lymphocytosis, influenza, exanthemata
    (ii) Bacterial: pyogenic infections in young children, convalescence from acute infections, pertussis, typhoid, brucellosis, TB, syphilis
    (iii) Protozoal: toxoplasmosis

2. Lymphatic leukaemia
3. Miscellaneous
    (i) Myasthenia gravis
    (ii) Thyrotoxicosis
    (iii) Hypopituitarism
    (iv) Carcinoma
    (v) Myelomatosis
4. Physiological in early childhood

Causes of eosinophilia (>440 x 10^6/l)
1. Allergy to food or drugs
2. Parasites: hookworm, tapeworm, hydatid, ascaris, bilharzia, strongyloides, filaria, trichina, etc.
3. Skin disease
    (i) Scabies
    (ii) Dermatitis herpetiformis
    (iii) Atopic eczema
    (iv) Erythema neonatorum
4. Hypereosinophilic syndrome
5. Bronchopulmonary eosinophilia (p. 38)
6. Eosinophilia-myalgia syndrome (L-tryptophan)
7. Post-infectious rebound
8. Blood dyscrasias, including eosinophilic leukaemia
9. Malignancy, especially Hodgkin's
10. Eosinophilic granuloma
11. Post-splenectomy
12. Rheumatoid disease with extra-articular involvement
13. Sarcoidosis

Causes of monocytosis (>800 x 10^6/l)
    Infectious
        Viral—Infectious mononucleosis
        Rickettsial—Rocky Mountain spotted fever
        Bacterial—*Listeria monocytogenes,* TB, brucellosis, typhoid
        Protozoal—Malaria, kala-azar, trypanosomiasis
2. Hodgkin's disease
3. Monocytic leukaemia

LYMPHADENOPATHY

CAUSES

1. **Infections**
    (i) Focal infection with regional lymphadenopathy, e.g. sepsis, TB, primary chancre
    (ii) HIV, e.g. persistent generalized lymphadenopathy
    (iii) Infectious mononucleosis
    (iv) Rubella
    (v) Secondary syphilis

    (vi) Toxoplasmosis
   (vii) Tropical infestation, e.g. filariasis

2. **Lymphoma**
    (i) Hodgkin's
   (ii) Non-Hodgkin's

3. **Leukaemia**
Usually lymphocytic

4. **Malignancy**
    (i) Metastases
   (ii) Reactive changes

5. **Miscellaneous**
    (i) Sarcoidosis
   (ii) Histiocytosis X (Langerhans cell)
   (iii) Chronic inflammatory skin disease
   (iv) Collagen vascular disease, e.g. RA, SLE
    (v) Anticonvulsant drugs
   (vi) Kikuchi's disease (with high fever)

HODGKIN'S DISEASE

Essential criteria for the histological diagnosis of Hodgkin's disease
1. Complete or partial destruction of the nodal architecture (reticulin stain)
2. Presence of abnormal reticulum cells
3. Presence of Sternberg–Reed giant cells

Clinical staging

Stage	Description
I	Disease limited to one anatomical region
II	(1) Disease limited to two contiguous anatomical regions on same side of the diaphragm
	(2) Disease in more than two anatomical regions or in two non-contiguous regions on same side of diaphragm
III	Disease on both sides of diaphragm but limited to involvement of lymph nodes, spleen and Waldeyer's ring
IV	Involvement of any tissue or organ other than lymph nodes, spleen or Waldeyer's ring

All stages are subclassified as A or B to indicate the absence or presence, respectively, of symptoms

CLASSIFICATION OF LEUKAEMIA

ACUTE ('Poorly differentiated')

1. Acute myeloid (AML)

Subdivided according to predominant cells
  (i) Myeloblastic
  (ii) Promyelocytic
  (iii) Myelocytic
  (iv) Myelomonocytic
  (v) Monocytic
  (vi) Erythro-leukaemia

2. Acute lymphoblastic (ALL)

  (i) Null cell (80%)
  (ii) T cell
  (iii) B cell

Distinguished from other types by
  a. peak incidence at 3–5yr
  b. better response to treatment, with long remission
  c. mature cells with normal morphology

CHRONIC ('Well-differentiated')

1. Myeloid

  (i) Chronic granulocytic (CGL)
      Most are Philadelphia chromosome positive. In the
      atypical juvenile form, Hb F is increased
  (ii) Chronic myelomonocytic (with high neutrophil count)
  (iii) Chronic monocytic (with normal or low neutrophil count)
  (iv) Neutrophilic (very rare)

2. Lymphocytic

  (i) Chronic lymphocytic (CLL)—usually B cells
  (ii) Chronic leukaemia with lymphoma
      e.g. Waldenstrom's macroglobulinaemia
          Follicular lymphoma
          Diffuse lymphocytic lymphoma
          Sézary syndrome (with pruritus, erythroderma and
          circulating Sézary T cells)
  (iii) Prolymphocytic leukaemia (characteristic vesicular cell—rare)
  (iv) Hairy cell leukaemia (atypical 'hairy' B cells)

MYELOPROLIFERATIVE DISEASES

1. Primary polycythaemia vera
2. Myelofibrosis
3. Thrombocythaemia
4. Erythroleukaemia (Di Guglielmo)

5. Atypical myeloproliferative disorders
   Some authorities now exclude leukaemia from the myeloproliferative disorders, although transitions can occur as follows:

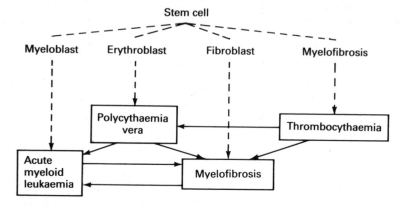

CAUSES OF POLYCYTHAEMIA

Absolute
1. Idiopathic PC Vera
2. Secondary
   (i) *Hypoxic*
      High altitude
      Cardiac or pulmonary disease
      Cerebral (decreased respiratory drive)
      Obesity (Pickwickian syndrome)
      Methaemoglobinaemia and sulphaemoglobinaemia
   (ii) *Erythropoietin*
      Cigarette smoking, even in absence of lung disease
      Kidney disease
      Carcinoma of liver
      Cerebellar haemangioblastoma
      Uterine myomata
      Virilizing syndromes
      Phaeochromocytoma
   (iii) *Benign familial*, due to abnormal Hb with either high
      oxygen affinity or excess methaemoglobin
   (iv) *Hypertransfusion*

Relative
1. Dehydration
2. 'Stress' polycythaemia (Gaisböck)
   Associated with hypertension, anxiety and high normal RBC
   mass or low normal plasma volume

SPLENOMEGALY

Causes
1. Infections
   - (i) Viral: infective hepatitis, infectious mononucleosis
   - (ii) Bacterial: septicaemia, SABE, TB, syphilis, brucellosis, typhoid
   - (iii) Rickettsial: typhus
   - (iv) Fungal: histoplasmosis
   - (v) Protozoal: malaria, kala-azar, trypanosomiasis
   - (vi) Parasitic: hydatid
2. Blood dyscrasia
   - (i) Leukaemia
   - (ii) Haemolytic anaemia
   - (iii) Myelofibrosis
   - (iv) Polycythaemia vera
   - (v) Occasionally in ITP, myelomatosis, megaloblastic anaemia and chronic Fe-deficiency anaemia
3. Malignant lymphomas
4. Miscellaneous
   - (i) Portal hypertension
   - (ii) Lipid storage disease
   - (iii) Benign tumours and cysts
   - (iv) Occasionally in SLE, sarcoidosis, amyloidosis, Rh arthritis, hyperthyroidism, etc.

Causes of a huge spleen

Chronic myeloid leukaemia
Myelofibrosis
Lymphocytic lymphoma
Malaria
Kala-azar
Gaucher's disease

In exams look for evidence of iliac bone biopsy as this suggests myelofibrosis

Causes of moderately large spleen

Above 6
+ Storage diseases
  Haemolytic anaemias
  Portal hypertension
  Leukaemias

Causes of a just palpable spleen

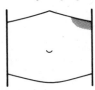

Above 10
+ all other causes of
splenomegaly (q.v.)

HYPERSPLENISM

(Reduction of one or more of the formed elements of the blood due to functional hyperactivity of the spleen)

Causes
1. Portal hypertension
2. Malignant lymphoma
3. Chronic lymphatic leukaemia or myelofibrosis, especially after repeated transfusions
4. Lipidoses (Gaucher's, Niemann–Pick's)
5. Sarcoidosis
6. Chronic infection
   TB, brucellosis, bacterial endocarditis
   Kala-azar and malaria
7. Rheumatoid disease (especially Felty's syndrome)
8. Red cell disorders
   Congenital, e.g. thalassaemia, spherocytosis
   Acquired, e.g. autoimmune haemolysis, paroxysmal nocturnal haemoglobinuria
9. Idiopathic

Common indications for splenectomy
1. Surgical, including trauma
2. Hereditary spherocytosis
3. Chronic ITP
4. Hypersplenism causing symptoms

Other indications
5. Acquired haemolytic anaemia
6. Acute ITP
7. Hereditary elliptocytosis
8. Myelofibrosis
9. Chronic lymphatic leukaemia
10. Malignant lymphomas
11. Thalassaemia major

HYPOSPLENISM

Causes
1. Splenectomy
2. Congenital
   (i)   Congenital absence
   (ii) Congenital cyanotic heart disease
3. Haematological
   (i)   Sickle cell disease
   (ii) Essential thrombocythaemia
   (iii) Fanconi's syndrome

4. Autoimmune
    (i)   Systemic lupus erythematosus
    (ii) Glomerulonephritis/vasculitis
    (iii) Rheumatoid arthritis
    (iv) Hashimoto's disease
    (v)   Graves' disease
5. Intestinal
    (i)   Coeliac disease (including dermatitis herpetiformis)
    (ii) Ulcerative colitis, Crohn's disease, tropical sprue, Whipple's disease
    (iii) Intestinal lymphangiectasia
6. Miscellaneous
    (i)   Splenic irradiation
    (ii) Amyloidosis
    (iii) Sarcoidosis
    (iv) Sézary's syndrome
    (v)   Chronic active hepatitis
    (vi) Thrombosis of splenic artery or vein
   (vii) Graft-versus-host disease
  (viii) Immunodeficiency
    (ix) Hypopituitarism

Complications (see also p. 74)
1. Susceptibility to infections (especially pneumococcal)
   Due to decreased polymorph phagocytosis and chemotaxis, and defective antibody responses
2. Increased autoantibody production
   May be due to impaired T suppressor cell activity
3. Increased risk of cardiac ischaemia
   Probably secondary to thrombocytosis and increased viscosity
4. Thrombosis
   Controversial—some studies have shown no increased risk

PLATELETS

Causes of thrombocytopenia ($<150 \times 10^9$/l)
1. *Decreased production*
    (i)   Marrow aplasia, e.g. drugs or toxins
    (ii) Marrow infiltration, e.g. leukaemia
    (iii) Uraemia
    (iv) Megaloblastic anaemia
    (v)   Alcoholism
    (vi) Viral infections, e.g. measles vaccination
2. *Decreased survival*
   Immunological
    (i)   Idiopathic thrombocytopenic purpura (ITP)

(ii) Drugs affecting platelets selectively, e.g. quinine, sulphonamides, thiazides, rifampicin, indomethacin, phenylbutazone, heparin

(iii) Blood transfusion with incompatible platelets

(iv) 'Secondary' thrombocytopenia—
   a. SLE
   b. Chronic lymphatic leukaemia
   c. Autoimmune haemolytic anaemia with ITP (Evans' syndrome)

Increased consumption
   (i) Disseminated intravascular coagulation (DIC) (p. 97)
   (ii) Thrombotic thrombocytopenic purpura (Moschcowitz's)
   (iii) Haemolytic-uraemic syndrome
   (iv) Large haemangiomata
   (v) Infections—R.M. Spotted Fever
                  Typhus
                  Bacterial endocarditis
                  Meningococcal septicaemia
                  Exanthemata
   (vi) Cardiopulmonary bypass
   (vii) Heparin therapy (in 1%)

3. *Sequestration*—Hypersplenism, hypothermia
4. *Dilution*—Massive transfusion of stored blood
5. *Loss*—Massive haemorrhage

In some conditions, e.g. uraemia and hypothermia, there may be several mechanisms

In neonates and children the following must also be considered:

1. Rare congenital disorders
   (i) Fanconi's aplastic anaemia (with multiple congenital anomalies)
   (ii) Familial thrombocytopenia
   (iii) Megakaryocyte aplasia
   (iv) Aldrich–Wiskott syndrome (with eczema and immunological deficiencies)
   (v) May Hegglin anomaly (with giant platelets)
   (vi) TAR syndrome (with absent radii)

2. Mothers with ITP, SLE or drug purpura

3. Viral or parasitic: Congenital rubella syndrome
                          Toxoplasmosis
                          Cytomegalic inclusion disease

4. Cyanotic congenital heart disease

5. Giant haemangioma

6. DIC

7. Exchange transfusion

Causes of qualitative platelet defects (i.e. platelet dysfunction)

A. *Congenital*
 1. Hereditary thrombasthenia (Glanzmann)
    Impaired platelet aggregation and clot retraction
 2. Congenital abnormalities of platelet release or adhesion
 3. Giant platelet syndrome (Bernard–Soulier)
 4. Associated with other hereditary disease
    (i) von Willebrand's disease, and some haemophilia
    (ii) Hermansky–Pudlak (with albinism)
    (iii) Chediak–Higashi (with abnormal granules in melanocytes
       and neutrophils)
    (iv) Cutis hyperelastica (Ehlers–Danlos)
    (v) Wiskott–Aldrich
    (vi) TAR syndrome (with absent radii)

B. *Acquired*
 1. Drugs
    (i) Aspirin
    (ii) Indomethacin
    (iii) Phenylbutazone
    (iv) Streptokinase
    (v) High MW dextran infusion
 2. Systemic diseases
    (i) Uraemia
    (ii) Liver disease
    (iii) Dysproteinaemia
    (iv) Scurvy
    (v) SLE
 3. Myeloproliferative disease, esp. thrombocythaemia (excessive
    platelets of abnormal morphology)
 4. Aplastic anaemia or leukaemia

Causes of thrombocytosis (Increased platelets, >400 x 10^9/l)
 1. Haemorrhage, surgery, trauma
 2. Splenectomy or splenic atrophy
 3. Myeloproliferative disorders, especially megakaryocytic
    leukaemia and haemorrhagic thrombocythaemia
 4. Chronic inflammatory disease
 5. Malignancy
 6. 'Rebound' after recovery from haemolysis or treatment of
    pernicious anaemia
 7. Chronic renal disease

Causes of thrombophilia

A. *Inherited*
 1. Antithrombin III deficiency
 2. Heparin cofactor II deficiency

3. Protein C deficiency: Purpura fulminans
                            Skin necrosis with warfarin therapy
4. Protein S deficiency
5. Dysfibrinogenaemia
6. Abnormalities in fibrinolysis

B. *Acquired*
 1. Malignant disease
 2. Anticardiolipin antibody (Lupus anticoagulant)
 3. Vasculitis
 4. Nephrotic syndrome
 5. Polycythaemia and essential thrombocythaemia
 6. Paraproteinaemia
 7. Chronic inflammatory disorders

Conditions predisposing to venous thrombosis

A. *Localized*
 1. Stasis (tight bandages, senility, immobility, etc.)
 2. Damaged vessel wall
     (i)   Infection
     (ii) Atheroma
     (iii) Trauma

B. *Generalized*
 1. Thrombophilia (p. 91)
 2. Prolonged bed rest
 3. Pregnancy and puerperium
 4. Oral contraceptives
 5. Sickle cell disorders
 6. Paroxysmal nocturnal haemoglobinuria
 7. Psoriasis
 8. Alcohol withdrawal
 9. Congestive heart failure
10. Chronic infection
11. Blood group A1
12. Family history of thrombosis

NB Cigarette smoking is a major risk factor for arterial thrombosis,
but may protect against venous thrombosis

ANTITHROMBIN III (AT III)

An important physiological inhibitor of thrombin and activated
clotting factor (Xa). Patients having major surgery with AT III levels
below 80% are at major risk of postoperative deep vein thrombosis

Causes of decreased AT III
1. Congenital familial deficiency
2. Liver disease
3. Disseminated intravascular disease
4. Postoperatively
5. Oral contraceptives

ANTICARDIOLIPIN ANTIBODY (ACA)

'Lupus anticoagulant' activity was first reported in patients with
SLE. The abnormality was a prolongation of the kaolin partial
thromboplastin time which was not corrected by the addition of
normal serum. The anticoagulant activity was subsequently shown
to be due to an anticardiolipin antibody (ACA), which paradoxically
predisposes to thrombosis. ACA also occurs in many patients who
do not have SLE

Clinical syndromes associated with ACA
1. Arterial or venous thromboses (may affect major vessels)
2. Recurrent abortion, often with areas of placental infarction
3. Neurological disorders
    (i) Cerebral thrombosis or vasoconstriction
    (ii) Optic neuritis
    (iii) Guillain Barré syndrome
    (iv) Chorea
    (v) Psychiatric changes
4. Thrombocytopenia
5. Livedo reticularis with 'stroke' and/or leg ulcers

VESSEL DEFECTS

Causes of bleeding due to defects of vessels or supportive tissues

A. *Acquired*
1. *Vasculitis* (p. 194), especially Henoch–Schönlein purpura and
   allergic vasculitis due to drugs
2. *Defect in connective tissue*
    (i) Senile purpura
    (ii) Cushing's disease or glucocorticoid therapy
    (iii) Scurvy (controversial, since platelets are defective)
3. *Amyloidosis* (primary and secondary)
4. *Anoxia*
    (i) Dysproteinaemia
    (ii) Fat embolism
5. *Infections*
    (i) Bacterial endocarditis
    (ii) Septicaemia
    (iii) Viral and rickettsial infections

6. *Dermatoses*
    (i)   Eczema
    (ii) Pigmented purpuric dermatosis (Schamberg, etc.)
    (iii) Drug-induced capillaropathy, especially carbromal
    (iv) Simple easy bruising
    (v)   Erythrocyte autosensitization ('psychogenic' purpura)

B. *Congenital*
   1. Hereditary haemorrhagic telangiectasia
   2. Hereditary capillary fragility
   3. Pseudo-xanthoma elasticum
   4. Cutis hyperelastica (Ehlers–Danlos)

COAGULATION

The coagulation cascade
Several factors (Fletcher, Fitzgerald, Passovoy) involved in the initial
phase of intrinsic coagulation have been described, but their role is
not fully understood
Factor XII is also involved in:
   1. activation of fibrinolysis
   2. conversion of kallikreinogen to kallikrein
   3. formation of plasma permeability factor

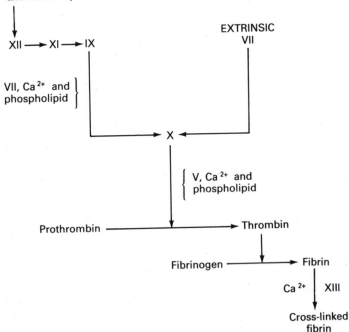

Blood coagulation factors

- I Fibrinogen
- II Prothrombin
- III Thromboplastin (tissue extract)
- IV (Ca^{2+})
- V Proaccelerin (labile)
- VI Accelerin (a hypothetical intermediate product)
- VII Proconvertin (stable)
- VIII Anti-haemophilic globulin
- IX Christmas factor
- X Stuart–Prower factor
- XI Plasma-thromboplastin antecedent (PTA)
- XII Hageman factor
- XIII Fibrin-stabilizing factor

Prekallikrein (Fletcher factor): deficiency is asymptomatic
Passovoy factor: deficiency resembles haemophilia
Vitamin K deficiency affects II, VII, IX and X

Factor VIII

Factor VIII has three components

1. VIII_c, necessary for coagulation, is measured by clotting assay
2. VIII_{vw}, necessary for platelet adhesion, is measured by ristocetin aggregation assay
3. VIII_{Ag}, which carries the active moieties, is measured by immunological assay

	Haemophilia A	*von Willebrand's*
VIII_c	Low	Low
VIII_{vw}	N	Low
VIII_{Ag}	N or High	N or Low

Platelets in von Willebrand's disease are probably not inherently defective, but only by virtue of the Factor VIII_{vw} deficiency

SCREENING TESTS FOR A BLEEDING DISORDER

1. **Blood count and film**
   To detect leukaemia and assess platelet number, size and shape

2. **Platelet count**
3. **Bleeding time** (with Duke's method, normal <7 min)
   Useful in diagnosis of von Willebrand's disease

4. **Hess test,** with sphygomomanometer cuff at c. 100 mmHg for 5 min (N<5 petechiae in a circle of 3 cm diameter)

5. **One-stage prothrombin time** (N 12–15 sec)—clotting time of citrated plasma to which brain emulsion (thromboplastin) and

calcium have been added
Tests the extrinsic system
Prolonged in
  (i) Deficiency of II, V, VII or X
  (ii) Severe fibrinogen deficiency
  (iii) Presence of some inhibitors, e.g. heparin or fibrin
       degradation products

6. **Activated partial thromboplastin time (APTT)** (N 30–45 sec)
   Tests the intrinsic system (especially VIII and IX)
   Uses kaolin in place of 'exposed collagen'

7. **Calcium thrombin time** (N 10–20 sec)
   Prolonged in
    (i) Fibrinogen deficiency
    (ii) Presence of some inhibitors, e.g. heparin

8. **Prothrombin consumption index**
   Very sensitive test which detects both platelet and coagulation
   abnormalities

9. **Fibrin degradation products**
   Increased in fibrinolysis
   Normal screening tests do not exclude vascular defects, e.g.
   senile purpura or mild coagulation factor deficiency, e.g. VIII
   (Haemophilia A) or IX (Haemophilia B)

Clinical feature	Coagulation disorder	Platelet disorder
Purpura	Rare	Common
Bruises	Single, deep	Multiple, superficial
Bleeding sites	Joints, muscles	Mucous membranes
Superficial cuts	Bleeding stops	Bleeding prolonged
Deep cuts	Bleeding continues despite pressure	Bleeding stops with pressure
Healing of cuts	Delayed	Normal

Results of tests in common bleeding disorders

	Prothrombin time	Partial thromboplastin time	Thrombin time	Platelet count
Liver disease	↑	↑	Usually N	N initially
Warfarin	↑	↑	N	N
Factor VII def.	↑	N	N	N
Haemophilia	N	↑	N	N
Christmas disease	N	↑	N	N
Heparin	↑	↑	↑	N
Disseminated intravascular coagulation	↑	↑	↑	↓

N = normal

CAUSES OF FIBRINOGEN DEFICIENCY (<1.5 g/l)

In many cases there are multiple causes

Acquired
1. *Impaired formation*, e.g. liver disease
2. *Increased consumption* ('disseminated intravascular coagulation', q.v.)
3. *Increased destruction* (excessive fibrinolysis)
   Usually secondary to 'disseminated intravascular coagulation'

Congenital
Very rare

DISSEMINATED INTRAVASCULAR COAGULATION

This is characterized by excessive formation of fibrinogen derivatives, usually due to increased proteolysis. There may be bleeding or thrombosis of any severity

Causes
1. 'Shock', esp. Gram neg. septicaemia and anaphylaxis
2. Other infections, e.g. TB, viral and fungal
3. Obstetric
   Premature placental separation
   Retention of dead fetus
   Amniotic embolism
   Fetal death due to Rh incompatibility
4. Major surgery, especially with extracorporeal shunts
5. Incompatible blood transfusion
6. Miscellaneous
   Leukaemia or carcinomatosis
   Liver, renal or prostatic disease

Pulmonary embolism
Snake venom
Trauma or burns
Hypothermia

Minimum laboratory criteria for diagnosis
At least 2 of the following:
1. Increased fibrin degradation products in serum
2. Decreased plasma fibrinogen
3. Prolonged thrombin clotting time
4. Positive ethanol gelation
In severe cases there may be a decrease in platelets, and factors II, V and VIII

Differential diagnosis of DIC

	Prothrombin time	Partial thromboplastin time	Thrombin time	Platelet count
DIC	↑↑	↑↑	↑↑	↓ or ↓↓
Massive stored blood transfusion	↑	↑	N	↓
Acute vitamin K deficiency	↑↑	↑	N	N
Haemophilia	N	↑↑	N	N
ITP	N	N	N	↓↓

↑ = increased
↑↑ = greatly increased
↓ = decreased
↓↓ = greatly decreased

CAUSES OF HYPOPROTHROMBINAEMIA

1. *Vitamin K deficiency*
   (i) Dietary deficiency (uncommon)
   (ii) Defective synthesis by intestinal bacteria, e.g. in neonates or after antibiotics
   (iii) Malabsorption, e.g. biliary obstruction
   (iv) Renal failure (probably multifactorial)
2. *Liver disease*
3. *Drugs*
   (i) Vitamin K antagonists
   (ii) Thiouracil, salicylates, etc.
4. *Carcinomatosis* (uncommon)
5. *Congenital* (very rare)

Conditions associated with circulating anticoagulants
 1. *Anticoagulants to AHG, etc.*
     (i)   Haemophilia (? due to repeated transfusions)
     (ii) Pregnancy, often with Rh incompatibility
     (iii) Malignancy
     (iv) Collagen-vascular disease
     (v)   Pemphigus
     (vi) Idiopathic
 2. *Heparin-like anticoagulants*
     (i)   Irradiation
     (ii) Cytotoxic therapy

COMPLICATIONS OF BLOOD TRANSFUSION

 1. *Febrile reactions*
     (i)   Pyrogens
     (ii) Leukocyte or platelet isoagglutinins
     (iii) Hypersensitivity to plasma
 2. *Allergic reactions*
 3. *Circulatory overload*
 4. Haemolysis. Red cells of either donor or recipient may be affected
     (i)   Blood group incompatibility
     (ii) Improper or overlong storage of donor blood
 5. *Reaction due to infected stored blood*
 6. *Disease transmission*
     (i)   Viral hepatitis (B and C), HIV, cytomegalovirus, Epstein–Barr virus, herpes simplex
     (ii) Syphilis
     (iii) Malaria, toxoplasmosis
     (iv) Brucellosis
 7. *Thrombophlebitis*
 8. *Air embolism*
 9. *Immunological sensitization by compatible blood,* especially Rhesus sensitization
10. *Transfusion siderosis*
11. *Complications of massive transfusion*
     (i)   Collapse due to cold blood
     (ii) Excess citrate (exaggerates bleeding tendency)
     (iii) Excess ammonia from stored blood (exaggerates precoma in cirrhotics)
     (iv) Excess potassium (exaggerates hyperkalaemia in uraemic patients)
     (v)   Thrombocytopenia
12. *Development of circulating anticoagulants,* e.g. AHG antibody

Neurology

BRAIN DEATH

Electroencephalography is not necessary for the diagnosis of brain death, but if an artificial life support system is to be withdrawn (e.g. for donation of organs for transplantation) the following tests should be performed by two doctors, one of whom should preferably be the consultant in charge of the case, and the tests may need to be repeated. The interval between the tests will depend on the primary pathology and the clinical course of the disease, and it might be as long as 24 hours. The body temperature should be not less than 35 °C before the diagnostic tests are performed.

Diagnostic tests for the confirmation of brain death
All brainstem reflexes are absent:
1. Pupils fixed and do not react to light
2. No corneal reflex
3. No vestibulo-ocular reflexes (using 20 ml of ice cold water in each external auditory meatus)
4. No motor responses in the cranial nerve distribution following adequate stimulation of any somatic area
5. No gag reflex to a suction catheter passed down the trachea
6. No respiratory movements occur when the patient is disconnected from the respirator for long enough to ensure a rise in arterial P_{CO_2} above 50 mmHg (threshold for stimulation of respiration). Patients with pre-existing chronic respiratory insufficiency will require special consideration

GLASGOW COMA SCALE

Used to monitor changes in level of consciousness

Eyes	Open	Spontaneously	4
		To verbal command	3
		To pain	2
	No response		1
Best motor response	To verbal command	Obeys	6
	To painful stimuli	Localizes pain	5
		Flexion—withdrawal	4
		Flexion—abnormal (decorticate rigidity)	3
		Extension (decerebrate rigidity)	2
		No response	1
Best verbal response		Oriented and converses	5
		Disoriented and converses	4
		Inappropriate words	3
		Incomprehensible sounds	2
		No response	1
Total			3–15

CAUSES OF COMA

1. *Head injury*
2. *Epilepsy*
3. *Drugs*
    Alcohol
    Hypnotics
    Carbon monoxide
    Aspirin
4. *Metabolic*
    Hyper- or hypo-glycaemia
    Uraemia
    Myxoedema
    Hepatic failure
    Hypoadrenalism
    Hypopituitarism
    Hypocapnia
    Electrolyte imbalance

5. *Vascular*
    Cerebral thrombosis, embolism, haemorrhage
    Hypertensive encephalopathy
    Causes of syncope (p. 14)
6. *Pressure effect*
    Space-occupying lesions
    Hydrocephalus
7. *Acute infection of CNS*
    Meningitis
    Encephalitis
    Abscess
8. *Acute systemic infection*
    Malaria
    Septicaemia
9. *Hysteria or hypnosis*
10. *Hyper-* or *hypo-thermia.*

CAUSES OF ASEPTIC MENINGITIS

A. Infection
1. Viral
2. Bacterial   Partially treated intracranial abscess or
                    empyema
                    Tuberculosis
3. Spirochaetes Leptospirosis, Lyme disease, syphilis, rickettsiae
4. Mycoplasma
5. Fungi   Histoplasma, coccidioidomycosis
6. Protozoal   Malaria, amoebae, trypanosomiasis
7. Helminths   Strongyloides, schistosomiasis

B. Others
1. Sarcoidosis
2. Whipple's disease
3. Molleret's meningitis
4. Vogt–Koyanagi–Harada syndrome
5. SLE, Behçet's disease
6. Neoplasm
7. Lead encephalopathy
8. Post-vaccination

HARMFUL EFFECTS OF ALCOHOL (ethanol and congeners)

1. *Social complications of intoxication or alcoholism*
2. *Physical complications of acute intoxication*
    e.g. accidents, coma, inhaled vomitus, Mallory–Weiss
    syndrome, 'hang-over'
3. *Neuropsychiatric*
    (i) Withdrawal syndromes

a. Tremulousness
b. Psychoses (paranoia, hallucinations, etc.)
c. Epilepsy (also pptd by hypoglycaemia)
d. Delirium tremens

(ii) Nutritional deficiency syndromes
a. Wernicke–Korsakoff syndrome
Ophthalmoplegia with nystagmus
Ataxia
Confusion and dullness
Amnesia and confabulation
b. Peripheral neuropathy (Wallerian degeneration)
c. Cerebellar degeneration
d. Central pontine myelinolysis (produces bulbar palsy)
e. Degeneration of corpus callosum
f. Retrobulbar neuropathy ('alcoholic amblyopia')

(iii) Toxic effects
a. Acute myositis after a drinking bout
b. Subacute myopathy (usually proximal)

(iv) Neurological effects of liver disease
a. Encephalopathy
b. Myelopathy (esp. after portacaval shunt)
c. Neuropathy (mild but not rare)

(v) Psychoses
Paranoia, hallucinations, morbid jealousy, fugue, increased
suicide risk, etc.

4. *Gastrointestinal*
(i) Acute gastritis and gastric ulcer
(ii) Fatty liver or alcoholic hepatitis
(iii) Cirrhosis
(iv) Pancreatitis
(v) Malabsorption
(vi) Increased risk of Ca. oesophagus

5. *Cardiac*
(i) Arrhythmia
(ii) Congestive cardiomyopathy
(iii) Hypertension
(iv) Beri-beri heart disease
(v) Cardiomyopathy due to cobalt additives in beer

6. *Haematological*
Diminished haemopoiesis (RBCs, WBCs and platelets) due to
dietary deficiency and toxic effect on marrow

7. *Metabolic*
(i) Obesity or malnutrition
(ii) Hypoglycaemia
(iii) Hyperlipaemia
(iv) Hyperuricaemia
(v) Increased cortisol production (pseudo-Cushing's)
(vi) Diuresis and electrolyte disturbance

(vii) Haemochromatosis
(viii) Porphyria cutanea tarda
8. *Increased incidence of infection,* esp. bacterial pneumonia, TB
9. *Skin*
   Association with psoriasis, esp. pustular (palmo-plantar)
10. *Effects on the fetus*
    (i) Increased risk of congenital defects
        a. Microcephaly
        b. Cardiac defect
        c. Growth deficiency
        d. Mental deficiency
    (ii) Increased perinatal mortality

CAUSES OF KORSAKOFF'S PSYCHOSIS

Alcoholism
Thiamine deficiency
Prolonged vomiting
Head injury
Cerebral anoxia
Cerebral tumours (primary or secondary)

CLASSIFICATION OF SPEECH DEFECTS

1. Dysphasia (disorder in use of symbols for communication whether spoken, heard, written or read)
2. Dysarthria (disorder of articulation)
3. Dysphonia (disorder of vocalization)
4. Dementia (intellectual deterioration)

Causes of dysphasia
1. Motor—due to lesion of inferior frontal gyrus of dominant frontal lobe (Broca's area)
2. Sensory—due to lesion of dominant temporoparietal cortex

Causes of dysarthria
1. *Bilateral upper motor-neurone (supranuclear) lesion of cranial nerves 9, 10 or 12 (Pseudo-bulbar palsy)*
   e.g. Cerebral ischaemia
        Motor neurone disease
        Multiple sclerosis
2. *Lower motor-neurone lesion of cranial nerves 9, 10 or 12 (Bulbar palsy)*
   e.g. Motor neurone disease
        Bulbar polio
        Medullary tumour
        Syringobulbia
        Guillain–Barré

3. *Basal ganglion lesions*
   e.g. Parkinsonism
       Choreoathetosis
       Hepatolenticular degeneration (Wilson's)
4. *Cerebellar lesions*
   e.g. Multiple sclerosis
       Toxins or drugs, especially alcohol
       Tumour
5. *Myasthenia gravis, facial muscular dystrophy and facial palsy*
6. *Oral lesions*
   e.g. False teeth
       Tongue-tie
       Cleft palate

Causes of dysphonia
1. Functional (hysteria)
2. Lesions of recurrent laryngeal nerve (Ca. bronchus, aortic aneurysm)
3. Vocal cord lesion (infection, tumour, etc.)

CAUSES OF DEMENTIA

Primary 'presenile' or 'senile' dementia
1. Idiopathic cerebral atrophy
2. Alzheimer's (senile plaques of extracellular amyloid, with surrounding neurofibrillary tangles)
3. Pick's (senile plaques, but neurofibrillary tangles are absent)
4. Creutzfeld–Jakob's transmissible dementia
5. Huntington's

Secondary

Intracranial
1. Infections
       Encephalitis, abscess or meningitis
       NB HIV (AIDS) and neurosyphilis, esp. GPI
2. Tumour, especially frontal
3. Vascular
     (i)   Subdural haematoma
     (ii) Atheroma
     (iii) Multiple small infarcts due to thromboemboli from heart or large arteries
     (iv) Vasculitis, e.g. SLE, Behçet's
     (v) Rarely, hypertension (Binswanger's disease)
4. Trauma (including repeated concussion in boxers and jockeys)
5. Multiple sclerosis and leukodystrophies
6. Neurolipidoses

7. Parkinsonism
8. Chronic epilepsy
9. Normal pressure hydrocephalus
10. Psychosis, e.g. schizophrenia, chronic depression

Extracranial
1. Metabolic
   (i)   Prolonged or recurrent anoxia or hypoglycaemia
   (ii) Chronic renal failure
   (iii) Hepatic failure
   (iv) Electrolyte imbalance
   (v)   Carcinomatous neuropathy (p. 129)
2. Endocrine
   (i)   Hypothyroidism
   (ii) Hypopituitarism
   (iii) Hypoadrenalism
   (iv) Hypo- or hyper-parathyroidism
3. Vitamin deficiency
   (i) B_{12} or folate
   (ii) Thiamine (esp. in alcoholics)
   (iii) Nicotinic acid (pellagra)
4. Drugs
   Barbiturates, cannabis, bromides, phenacetin, propranolol
5. Toxins
   Alcohol, lead, manganese, arsenic, aluminium (renal dialysis), etc.

CAUSES OF SEVERE AMNESIA

1. *Thiamine deficiency*
   (i)   Alcohol (Korsakoff syndrome)
   (ii) Dietary deficiency
   (iii) Hyperemesis gravidarum
   (iv) Gastric cancer
2. *Vascular*
   (i)   Bilateral thalamic infarcts
   (ii) Posterior cerebellar artery blockage
3. *Metabolic*
   Anoxia, hypoglycaemia, severe epilepsy, chronic sedative abuse, Halcion
4. *Infection* (temporal lobe damage)
   (i)   Meningitis, esp. TB
   (ii) Encephalitis, esp. herpes simplex
5. *Tumour or trauma* (including surgery and radiotherapy)
6. *Alzheimer's disease*
7. *Transient global amnesia* (may be transient ischaemic attack)

NEUROLOGICAL MANIFESTATIONS OF AIDS

1. *Functional*
   Anxiety, depression, etc. which may lead to suicide
2. *Primary HIV infection*
   (i)   Acute encephalopathy at time of seroconversion:
         May be EEG changes and epilepsy
   (ii) Chronic AIDS-dementia complex
         Occurs eventually in at least 60% of AIDS cases
   (iii) Vacuolar myelopathy
3. *Opportunistic infection*
   Toxoplasmosis, Cryptococcus, Listeria, etc.
   Progressive multifocal leucoencephalopathy
   Neurosyphilis
   Tuberculosis
   CMV encephalitis
4. *Neoplasm*
   Primary lymphoma or metastatic non-Hodgkin's
5. *Other*
   CMV retinitis
   Cranial or peripheral neuropathy
   Radiculopathy (Herpes zoster or CMV)
   Myalgia or myopathy

CAUSES OF EPILEPSY

1. *Idiopathic* (including genetic factors)
2. *Focal lesions*
   (i)   Birth injury
   (ii)   Tumour, esp. meningioma
   (iii) Trauma, scar
   (iv)   Vascular
          Angiomatous malformation
          Cerebral ischaemia or infarct
          Acute hypertension
   (v)   Infectious
          Encephalitis or meningitis
          Abscess or tuberculoma
          Neurosyphilis
          Hydatid or cysticercosis
   (vi)   Primary dementias (p. 105)
   (vii) Other neurological disease
          Multiple sclerosis, leukodystrophies
          Tuberous sclerosis (epiloia)
3. *Metabolic*
   (i)   Anoxia
   (ii) Hypoglycaemia
   (iii) Hypocalcaemia

  (iv)   Alkalosis
   (v)   Water intoxication
  (vi)   Uraemia
 (vii)   Hepatic coma
(viii)   Lipidoses (Tay–Sachs)
  (ix)   Drugs and chemicals
             Nikethamide, lignocaine
             Lead poisoning
             Cocaine
             Ether
             Withdrawal of alcohol or barbiturates
   (x)   Pyrexia, especially in children

CAUSES OF INTRACEREBRAL CALCIFICATION

1. Congenital toxoplasmosis
2. Tuberous sclerosis
3. Sturge–Weber syndrome
4. Craniopharyngioma
5. Tuberculosis
6. Old haematoma or healed abscess
7. Pineal gland (normal)
8. Hypoparathyroidism and pseudohypoparathyroidism

CAUSES OF DISSEMINATED CNS LESIONS

1. Multiple sclerosis
2. Meningovascular syphilis
3. Multiple infarcts
4. Multiple metastases
5. Subacute combined degeneration
6. Tabes dorsalis
7. Friedreich's ataxia
8. Neuromyelitis optica
9. Diffuse sclerosis
10. Progressive multifocal leukoencephalopathy

MECHANISMS OF HEADACHE PRODUCTION

1. *Skeletal muscle contraction*, e.g. 'tension' headache
2. *Referred pain*, e.g. disease of eyes, ears, sinuses, cervical spine
3. *Arterial dilatation*
    (i)   Intracranial, e.g. systemic infections, hypertension, nitrites, anoxia, 'hang-over', post-ictal, concussion
   (ii)   Extracranial, e.g. migraine

4. *Traction on arteries*, e.g. raised IC pressure (haemorrhage, tumour, etc.)
5. *Dilatation or traction on venous sinuses*, e.g. postlumbar puncture
6. *Inflammation*
   (i) Intracranial, e.g. meningitis
   (ii) Extracranial, e.g. giant-cell arteritis
7. *Psychogenic*

CAUSES OF HYDROCEPHALUS IN THE ADULT

1. Posterior fossa tumour
2. Subarachnoid haemorrhage
3. Head injury
4. Post-meningitis
5. Colloid cyst of third ventricle
6. Normal pressure hydrocephalus
7. Papilloma of the choroid plexus

CAUSES OF CATARACT

1. *Senility*
2. *Endocrine*
   Diabetes mellitus
   Hypoparathyroidism and pseudohypoparathyroidism
   Corticosteroid therapy
   Cretinism
3. *Hereditary and congenital conditions*
   Rubella syndrome
   Atopic eczema
   Down's syndrome
   Hepatolenticular degeneration
   Galactosaemia
   Dystrophia myotonica
   Oculocerebrorenal syndrome (Lowe)
   Laurence–Moon–Biedl (retinitis pigmentosa, polydactyly, obesity, hypogonadism, mental retardation)
   Refsum's (retinitis pigmentosa, deafness, ataxia, neuropathy)
4. *Secondary to ocular diseases*
   Glaucoma
   Ophthalmitis
   Degenerative myopia
   Retinal detachment
   Trauma
5. *Heat and irradiation*

CAUSES OF UVEITIS

(Uveal tract = iris, ciliary body and choroid)
1. *Miscellaneous systemic disease*
   (i)   Ankylosing spondylitis
   (ii) Reiter's disease
   (iii) Sarcoidosis
   (iv) Ulcerative colitis
   (v)   Rheumatoid disease, esp. Still's
   (vi) Behçet's disease (esp. in Turkey and Japan)
2. *Infections*
   (i)   Bacterial: TB
   (ii) Spirochaetal: Sy, relapsing fever, Weil's disease
   (iii) Fungal: histoplasmosis (in USA)
   (iv) Protozoal: malaria, toxoplasmosis
   (v)   Nematode larvae: toxocara of dog and cat
3. *Secondary to ocular disease*
   (i)   Ophthalmitis
   (ii) Trauma
4. *Idiopathic*

CAUSES OF RETINAL HAEMORRHAGE

1. Diabetes mellitus
2. Hypertension
3. Raised IC pressure
4. Retinal vein thrombosis
5. Trauma and retinal detachment
6. Arteritis (PN, cranial arteritis, etc.)
7. Subarachnoid haemorrhage
8. Severe anaemia, especially PA
9. Bleeding diathesis—defect in platelets (esp. leukaemia), vessels or coagulation factors

CAUSES OF ANGIOID STREAKS

1. Pseudoxanthoma elasticum
2. Sickle-cell disease
3. Ehlers–Danlos syndrome
4. Paget's disease of bone

CAUSES OF SUDDEN BLINDNESS

Ocular:
1. Trauma
2. Vitreous haemorrhage, especially in diabetics
3. Retinal detachment
4. Welding lights, etc.

5. Acute glaucoma
6. Embolism or spasm of retinal artery
7. Thrombosis of retinal vein
8. Acute optic neuritis, esp. cranial arteritis and methyl alcohol poisoning

Cerebral:
1. Cerebral infarct, haemorrhage or trauma
2. Hypertensive encephalopathy
3. Migraine
4. Acute hydrocephalus, esp. in children
5. Transient 'blackout', e.g. vasovagal
6. Hysteria

DRUG-INDUCED EYE DISEASE

1. **Eyelids**
   Pigmentation—chlorpromazine
   Eczema—topical chloramphenicol
   Angio-oedema—penicillin

2. **Conjunctiva and cornea**
   Punctate deposits—chloroquine, chlorpromazine, amiodarone
   Stevens–Johnson syndrome—sulphonamides
   Oculomucocutaneous syndrome—practolol

3. **Uvea** (iris, ciliary body and choroid)
   Blurred vision—anticholinergics
   Glaucoma—anticholinergics, antihistamines, antiparkinsonian
                    drugs

4. **Lens**
   Transient myopia—tetracycline, sulphonamide, acetazolamide
   Cataract—cholinesterase inhibitors, glucocorticoids,
               phenothiazines

5. **Retina**
   Retinopathy—chloroquine and derivatives,
                  phenothiazines, esp. thioridazine

6. **Optic nerve**
   Neuropathy
      (i) Neurotoxic—antituberculous drugs (isoniazid,
                        streptomycin, ethambutol)
     (ii) Ischaemic—quinine
    (iii) Nutritional—penicillamine (pyridoxine deficiency)

CRANIAL NERVE SUPPLY

1. *Olfactory*   Smell
2. *Optic*   Vision
3. *Oculomotor*
   (i)   All ocular muscles, except superior oblique and lateral rectus
   (ii)   Ciliary muscle
   (iii) Sphincter pupillae
   (iv)   Levator palpebrae superioris
4. *Trochlear*   Superior oblique muscle
   NB Tested by asking patient to look down and *inwards*
5. *Trigeminal*
   (i)   Sensory for face, cornea, sinuses, nasal mucosa, teeth, tympanic membrane and anterior two-thirds of tongue
   (ii)   Motor to muscles of mastication
6. *Abducens*   Lateral rectus muscle
7. *Facial*
   (i)   Motor to scalp and facial muscles of expression
   (ii)   Taste in anterior two-thirds of tongue (via chorda tympani)
   (iii) Nerve to stapedius muscle
8. *Auditory*   Auditory and vestibular components
9. *Glossopharyngeal*
   (i)   Sensory for posterior one-third of tongue, pharynx and middle ear
   (ii)   Taste fibres for posterior one-third of tongue
   (iii) Motor to middle constrictor of pharynx and stylopharyngeus
10. *Vagal*
   (i)   Motor to soft palate, larynx and pharynx (from nucleus ambiguus)
   (ii)   Sensory and motor for heart, respiratory passages and abdominal viscera (from dorsal nucleus)
11. *Spinal accessory*
   (i)   Motor to sternomastoid and trapezius
   (ii)   Accessory fibres to vagus
12. *Hypoglossal*   Motor to tongue and hyoid bone depressors

PATTERNS OF VISUAL FIELD LOSS

1. **Concentric diminution ('tunnel vision')**
   e.g. glaucoma

2. **Central scotoma**
   e.g. retinal disease involving macula, retrobulbar neuritis

3. **Complete field loss in one eye**
   e.g. optic nerve lesion

4. **Bitemporal hemianopia**
   e.g. pituitary tumour

5. **Homonymous hemianopia**
   e.g. tract lesions posterior to chiasma

6. **Quadrantic hemianopia**
   e.g. temporal lobe tumours for superior quadrant
   parietal lobe tumours for inferior quadrant

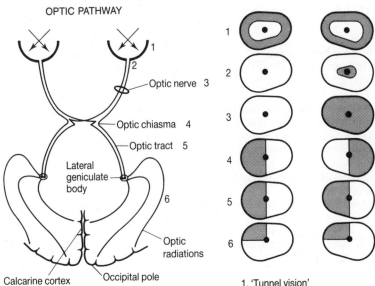

OPTIC PATHWAY

Optic nerve 3
Optic chiasma 4
Optic tract 5
Lateral geniculate body
Optic radiations
Calcarine cortex
Occipital pole

1. 'Tunnel vision'
2. Central scotoma
3. Complete field loss in one eye
4. Bitemporal hemianopia
5. Homonymous hemianopia
6. Quadrantic hemianopia

Causes of concentric diminution ('tunnel vision')
1. Glaucoma
2. Retinal disease, e.g. retinitis pigmentosa and choroidoretinitis
3. Papilloedema
4. Some types of optic atrophy, e.g. tabes dorsalis
5. Bilateral lesions of anterior calcarine cortex
6. Acute ischaemia, e.g. migraine
7. Hysteria

Causes of central scotoma
1. Retinal disease involving macula
2. Retrobulbar neuritis (MS and Leber's optic atrophy)
3. Optic atrophy due to compression, toxins or B_{12} deficiency
4. Lesions of occipital pole (e.g. trauma)

Causes of bitemporal hemianopia
Central chiasmal lesions
1. Pituitary or perisellar tumour (e.g. craniopharyngioma or meningioma)
2. Inflammatory, vascular or traumatic lesions (e.g. aneurysm of anterior communicating artery)

Binasal hemianopia
Very rare, being produced by bilateral lesions confined to the uncrossed optic fibres

Causes of homonymous hemianopia
Optic tract lesions—cerebral infarction or tumour may produce a hemianopia which bisects the macula
Occipital cortex infarct

Causes of homonymous hemianopia with ipsilateral central scotoma
Lesions of lateral part of optic chiasma which also affect the optic nerve
1. Pituitary tumour
2. Aneurysm of ant. communicating artery
3. Sphenoidal wing meningioma

Causes of homonymous quadrantanopia
Anteriorly placed lesions of the optic radiation, especially temporal lobe tumours. More posterior lesions of the optic radiation become more hemianopic
NB Retinal lesions (e.g. detachment, retinal arterial or venous occlusion) tend to respect the horizontal meridian

CAUSES OF OPTIC ATROPHY
1. *Glaucoma*
2. *Retinal lesions*
   Choroidoretinitis
   Intraocular haemorrhage, etc.
3. *Optic neuritis* (retrobulbar neuritis) (q.v.)
4. *Chronic papilloedema*

5. *Pressure on optic nerve*
   Tumour
   Aneurysm
   Paget's disease
6. *Division of optic nerve*
   Surgery
   Trauma

CAUSES OF OPTIC NEURITIS

1. *Ischaemia,* e.g. cranial arteritis
2. *Demyelinating disease*
   Multiple sclerosis
   Leukodystrophies
3. *Infective*
   Local: retinitis, periostitis, meningitis
   Systemic: syphilis, toxoplasmosis, typhoid fever
4. *Toxins*
   Methyl alcohol
   Lead
   Benzene
   Tobacco (defect in cyanide detoxication)
   Clioquinol (subacute myelo-optic neuropathy)
5. *Metabolic*
   Diabetes mellitus
   B_{12} deficiency
   Tropical ataxic neuropathy (cassava diet)
   Severe anaemia esp. haemorrhage
6. Behçet's disease
7 *Hereditary degenerations*
   e.g. Leber's, Friedreich's ataxia

CAUSES OF PAPILLOEDEMA

1. *Raised intracranial pressure* (q.v.)
2. *Arterial hypertension*
3. *Optic neuritis* (papillitis)
4. *Obstructed retinal venous drainage*
   (i) Tumour
   (ii) Thrombosis of central retinal vein
   (iii) Cavernous sinus thrombosis
5. *Miscellaneous rare causes*
   (i) Hypercapnia
   (ii) Exophthalmos
   (iii) SABE
   (iv) Hypoparathyroidism
   (v) Sudden or severe anaemia
   (vi) Lead poisoning

Papilloedema without papillitis tends to produce a large blind spot but normal visual acuity

Papillitis (Retrobulbar neuritis) tends to produce a large central scotoma with poor visual acuity, and pain on eye movement

Causes of raised intracranial pressure
1. Intracranial mass or infection
2. Obstructed c.s.f. flow
3. Hypertensive encephalopathy
4. Hypercapnia (CO_2 retention)
5. Pseudo-tumour cerebri
   (i)   Thrombosis of intracranial venous sinuses
   (ii) Many rare causes, e.g. oral contraceptives, vitamin A poisoning, retinoids, tetracycline

3rd cranial nerve (oculomotor) palsy
1. Marked ptosis
2. Eye abducted and depressed
3. Pupil **dilated** and completely nonreactive
   More often partial than complete, especially with lesions near the nucleus

Causes of oculomotor palsy
1. Aneurysm of posterior communicating artery
2. Tumours
3. Brain stem CVA

Cervical sympathetic paralysis (Horner's)
1. Mild ptosis
2. Enophthalmos
3. Pupil **constricted** with no reaction to shading
4. Reduced sweating on ipsilateral half of head and neck
5. Abolition of ciliospinal reflex
NB Everything gets 'smaller'

CERVICAL SYMPATHETIC PATHWAY TO THE EYE
1. Midbrain (superior colliculus)
2. Tectospinal tract (adjacent to lateral spinothalamic tract)
3. C8, T1 and 2 ventral roots
4. Cervical sympathetic trunk
5. Internal carotid and cavernous nerve plexus
6. Ophthalmic division of the trigeminal nerve

CAUSE OF PTOSIS
1. Congenital
2. Oculomotor nerve lesion

3. Cervical sympathetic lesion (Horner's)
4. Myasthenia gravis
5. Myopathy
6. Tabes dorsalis
7. Hysteria
Exclude congenital microphthalmos, contralateral exophthalmos

CAUSES OF MYDRIASIS (abnormally large pupil)

1. *Oculomotor nerve lesions*
   Characterized by
   (i)   Marked ptosis
   (ii) Large regular pupil fixed to light and accommodation
   (iii) External ophthalmoplegia (eye looks down and out)
2. *Parasympathetic paralysis,* e.g. atropine (acts via oculomotor nerve)
3. *Sympathetic stimulation* (e.g. adrenaline or cocaine)
   Pupils react normally to light and accommodation
4. *Optic nerve lesion*
   Pupil reacts sluggishly to direct light, but normally to consensual light and accommodation
5. *Lesions of eye* such as iritis, cataract or vitreous haemorrhage
6. *Deep coma*
7. *Myotonic pupil* (Holmes–Adie)

SQUINTS

Concomitant squint
Due to increased tone in one ocular muscle compared with its synergist. Usually congenital, but may follow an exanthem. Occurs in all neonates

Features
1. Both eyes have full movement if tested separately
2. No diplopia

Paralytic squint
Due to lesions of 3rd, 4th or 6th cranial nerves. Usually causes diplopia

Features
1. 'False' image is always peripheral
2. 'False' image is seen by affected eye
3. Separation of images is maximal in direction of action of affected muscle

EYE MOVEMENTS

With the eye turned *laterally* the *elevators* and depressors are the *superior* and inferior recti respectively
With the eye turned *medially* the *elevators* and depressors are the *inferior* and superior obliques respectively

THE ANATOMY OF THE FACIAL NERVE

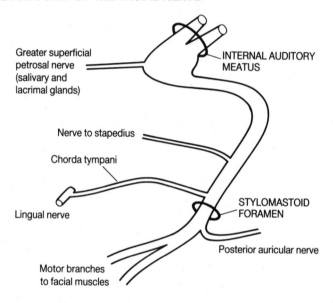

Greater superficial petrosal nerve (salivary and lacrimal glands)

INTERNAL AUDITORY MEATUS

Nerve to stapedius

Chorda tympani

Lingual nerve

STYLOMASTOID FORAMEN

Posterior auricular nerve

Motor branches to facial muscles

Hints on localization of lesion in facial paralysis
1. Associated lesions may help
   e.g. Ipsilateral 6th nerve palsy suggests brainstem
       5th and 8th nerve lesions suggest cerebellopontine angle
       Hyperacusis (n. to stapedius) and loss of taste (lingual n.)
       suggest bony canal
2. Paresis of frontalis muscle indicates a nuclear or infranuclear lesion
3. In supranuclear lesions emotional facial movements are occasionally retained

NB *Exclude myasthenia gravis and facial myopathy. They usually produce bilateral weakness, with ptosis*

Causes of bilateral L. M. N. facial paralysis
1. Guillain–Barré syndrome
2. Motor neurone disease
3. Sarcoidosis
4. Poliomyelitis
5. Post-meningitis
6. Bilateral acoustic neuromas
7. Cephalic tetanus

Causes of facial pain
1. Disease of teeth, sinuses, ear, nose or throat
2. Trigeminal neuralgia
3. Post-herpetic neuralgia
4. Migrainous neuralgia ('cluster' headache)
5. Aneurysm of post. communicating or int. carotid artery
6. Cranial arteritis
7. Raeder's paratrigeminal syndrome—Severe retro-orbital pain succeeded by ipsilateral miosis and ptosis
8. Superior orbital fissure syndrome—Boring retro-orbital pain and paresis of cranial nerves 3, 4, 5 and 6
9. Causalgia from partial 5th n. lesions
10. 'Atypical facial pain'—Constant, nagging deep pain not corresponding to any anatomical sensory distribution
11. Temporomandibular arthritis
12. Myocardial ischaemia (rarely)

Ramsay–Hunt syndrome (geniculate herpes zoster)
1. Vesicles on auricle or anterior fauces
2. Pain in ear and mastoid region
3. Ipsilateral taste loss in anterior two-thirds tongue
4. Facial paresis or spasm
5. Deafness or dizziness
6. Hyperacusis (paralysis of n. to stapedius)

CAUSES OF NYSTAGMUS
1. Physiological, e.g. optokinetic
2. Errors of refraction and macular lesions
3. Weakness of ocular muscles
4. Lesion of cranial nerves 3, 4 or 6
5. Brain stem lesions
6. Cerebellar lesions
7. Vestibular lesions
8. High cervical cord lesions
9. Idiopathic or congenital

DEAFNESS

CAUSES OF DEAFNESS

A. Conduction deafness
1. Wax or foreign-body
2. Eustachian obstruction
3. Otitis media
4. Otosclerosis
5. Paget's disease

B. Nerve deafness
1. Traumatic:
    (i) Chronic exposure to loud noise
    (ii) Fracture of petrous temporal bone
2. Infective:
    (i) Congenital syphilis
    (ii) Rubella syndrome
    (iii) Mumps, influenza
3. Toxic:
    (i) Aspirin, quinine
    (ii) Antibiotics, e.g. streptomycin, neomycin
    (iii) Tobacco, alcohol
4. Degenerative:
    Presbyacusis
5. Tumour, e.g. acoustic neuroma
6. Brain-stem lesions (rarely)
7. Rare familial syndromes

RINNE'S TEST

The ability to hear a tuning fork through air and through the mastoid process are compared. In *normal* people and in *nerve* deafness the air conducted sound is louder, whereas in conduction deafness it is softer

WEBER'S TEST

The base of the fork is placed on the centre of the forehead; in *nerve* deafness the note is heard in the *normal* ear, whereas in conduction deafness it is heard in the deaf ear

SOME CAUSES OF 'GIDDINESS'
1. True vertigo (p. 121)
2. Hypotension or hypertension
3. Anaemia

4. Intracranial hypertension
5. Hypoglycaemia
6. Epileptic aura
7. Migraine
8. Psychogenic

CAUSES OF VERTIGO

1. Vestibular lesions
   (i) Physiological
   (ii) Labyrinthitis
   (iii) Menière's
   (iv) Drugs, e.g. quinine, salicylates
   (v) Otitis media
   (vi) Motion sickness
   (vii) 'Benign post-traumatic positional vertigo'
2. Vestibular nerve lesions
   (i) Acoustic neuroma
   (ii) Drugs, e.g. streptomycin
   (iii) Vestibular neuronitis
3. Brain stem, cerebellar or temporal lobe lesions
   (i) Pontine infarction or haemorrhage
   (ii) Vertebrobasilar insufficiency
   (iii) Basilar artery migraine
   (iv) Disseminated sclerosis
   (v) Tumours
   (vi) Syringobulbia
   (vii) Temporal lobe epilepsy

CAUSES OF TRANSIENT FOCAL CEREBRAL ISCHAEMIC ATTACKS (TIA)

1. Emboli from heart or neck vessels
2. Mechanical effects
   (i) Cervical spondylosis
   (ii) Subclavian steal (proximal subclavian stenosis)
   (iii) Shunts
3. Increased arterial resistance, e.g. hypertension or migraine
4. Hypotension
5. Increased blood viscosity, e.g. polycythaemia
6. Anaemia

BASAL ARTERIES OF THE BRAIN

Anatomy of the circle of Willis

The anterior and middle cerebral arteries arise from the internal carotids, and the posterior from the basilar

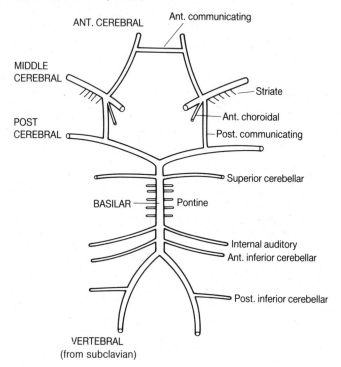

ANT. CEREBRAL   Ant. communicating

MIDDLE CEREBRAL

Striate

POST CEREBRAL

Ant. choroidal

Post. communicating

Superior cerebellar

BASILAR — Pontine

Internal auditory
Ant. inferior cerebellar

Post. inferior cerebellar

VERTEBRAL
(from subclavian)

CAUSES OF CEREBRAL INFARCTION

1. Atheroma of intra- or extracranial arteries
2. Cerebral emboli:
   (i) Atrial fibrillation
   (ii) Myocardial infarct
   (iii) Bacterial endocarditis
3. Cerebral ischaemia due to severe hypotension
4. Cerebral arterial spasm, e.g. migraine or following subarachnoid haemorrhage
5. Hypoxia, e.g.
   (i) Cardiac arrest
   (ii) Carbon monoxide poisoning
   (iii) Pulmonary emboli

6. Arteritis, e.g. collagen-vascular disease
7. Cerebral thrombosis, e.g. due to polycythaemia
8. Dissecting aortic aneurysm involving the carotid artery
9. Ligation of carotid artery for intracranial aneurysm

Features of post. inf. cerebellar artery thrombosis
1. Sudden onset of severe vertigo
2. Ipsilateral cerebellar ataxia, with nystagmus to side of lesion
3. Contralateral sensory loss of trunk and limbs to pain and temperature
4. Ipsilateral involvement of 5th to 8th nerves
5. Bulbar palsy
6. Ipsilateral cervical sympathetic paralysis
NB The occlusion may be transient

SPINAL CORD

Transverse section

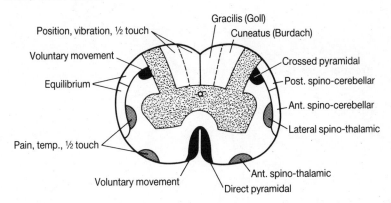

Tendon reflexes
Ankle	S 1, 2
Knee	L 3, 4
Biceps	C 5
Supinator	C 5, 6
Triceps	C 7

Superficial reflexes
Cremasteric	L 1, 2
Anal	S 3, 4
Plantar	S 1
Abdominal	T 8 to 12

Myotomes worth remembering

C6—Biceps, brachioradialis, radial extensors of wrist
C7—Triceps, ulnar extensors of wrist, finger extensors
C8—Finger flexors
L4—Quadriceps femoris
L5—Extensor hallucis longus
S1—Plantar flexors

Dermatomes of head and neck

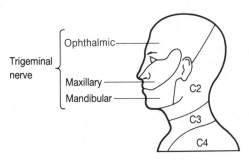

Dermatomes in the upper limb

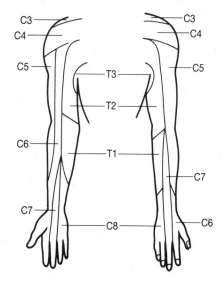

Dermatomes in the lower limb

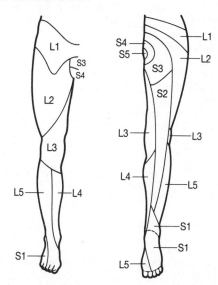

Nerve supply of diaphragm
Phrenic n. (C 3, 4, 5) descends under cover of sternomastoid m., passes in front of subclavian artery, then descends vertically in front of root of lung and passes between pericardium and mediastinal pleura to diaphragm. The diaphragm is also innervated peripherally by the lower 7 intercostal nerves

Course of recurrent laryngeal nerves (RLN)
Right RLN arises from vagus in the neck and winds backwards round first part of R subclavian artery. *Left* RLN arises from vagus in the superior mediastinum and winds backwards round arch of aorta. Both nerves then ascend between trachea and oesophagus and supply all muscles of larynx except cricothyroid
   Bilateral paralysis causes stridor ('cadaveric' cords)
   Unilateral paralysis causes dysphonia with 'bovine' cough

Causes of cord compression
  1. *Vertebral*
      (i)   Congenital bony anomaly
      (ii) Trauma
      (iii) Vertebral collapse
      (iv) Disc prolapse, spondylolisthesis, spondylosis
      (v)   Neoplasm (primary or secondary)
      (vi) Paget's
      (vii) Infection—TB or pyogenic

2. *Extradural*
   (i)   Hodgkin's, leukaemic infiltrate or metastases
   (ii) Abscess
   (iii) Cyst
3. *Intradural extramedullary*
   (i)   Neoplasm (meningioma, neurofibroma)
   (ii) Arachnoiditis
   (iii) Arachnoid cyst
4. *Intramedullary*
   (i)   Neoplasm, esp. glioma
   (ii) Cyst or syringomyelia
   (iii) Haematomyelia

Causes of paraplegia
1. Hereditary spastic paraplegia
2. Cerebral birth injury
3. Trauma
4. Cord compression—intra- or extramedullary (p. 125)
5. Multiple sclerosis
6. Transverse myelitis
7. Spinal artery occlusion, including meningovascular syphilis
8. Syringomyelia
9. Motor neurone disease
10. Poliomyelitis
11. Sub-acute combined degeneration
12. Guillain–Barré (Landry's ascending paralysis)
13. Friedreich's ataxia; familial spastic paraplegia, etc.
14. Sagittal sinus thrombosis
15. Midline precentral meningioma
16. Hysteria

Causes of dissociated anaesthesia (Loss of pain and temperature, but preservation of other sensation)
1. *Central cord lesion* affecting the crossing fibres, e.g. syringomyelia
2. *Cord hemisection* (*Brown–Séquard*)
   e.g. compression or intramedullary neoplasm
      Features
         (i)   LMN lesion at level of lesion
         (ii) UMN lesion below level of lesion
         (iii) Ipsilateral loss of position, vibration and touch
         (iv) Contralateral loss of pain and temperature
3. *Lesions of lateral medulla*
   e.g. posterior-inferior cerebellar thrombosis or syringobulbia

NEUROLOGICAL CONTROL OF BLADDER FUNCTION

Normal bladder capacity is 300–400 ml and larger volumes should stimulate the desire to micturate. Afferent fibres travel via parasympathetic nerves to spinal 'micturition centre' (S 2, 3, 4) and bladder contraction is initiated by parasympathetic efferents. The spinal 'micturition centre' is normally inhibited by higher motor centre, which bombard it with facilitatory impulses when micturition begins, so that the bladder empties completely

TYPES OF DYSFUNCTION

1. **Lack of normal inhibition**
   Frequency with small volumes
   Occurs in anxiety, cold weather, etc.

2. **Atonic bladder**
   Distended bladder with overflow, but no desire to micturate
   Occurs with sensory neuropathy, e.g. diabetes mellitus, tabes dorsalis

3. **Automatic bladder**
   Bladder empties partially when volume of about 250 ml is reached, but without desire to micturate
   Occurs with cord section above S 2, 3, 4

4. **Autonomous bladder**
   Large residual urine volume, with weak uncoordinated bladder contractions but no desire to micturate. Occurs with LMN cord lesions at S 2, 3, 4 level
   Unilateral neurological lesions may cause either frequency with small volumes or a large hypotonic bladder with residual urine after micturition

PERIPHERAL NERVES

Nerve supply to muscles of front of forearm

Ulnar nerve supplies
   1. Flexor carpi ulnaris
   2. Half of flexor digitorum profundus
Median nerve supplies all the rest

Nerve supply to short muscles of hand
Median nerve supplies
   1. Lateral two lumbricals
   2. Opponens pollicis
   3. Abductor pollicis brevis
   4. Flexor pollicis brevis

Mnemonic—'LOAF'
Ulnar nerve supplies all the rest
Abductor pollicis brevis is paralysed in T1 root lesions but not in ulnar nerve lesions

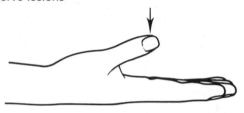

To test abductor pollicis brevis the thumb is moved vertically against resistance, with the hand supine

Causes of wasting of small muscles of hand
1. *Cord lesions at T1 level*
   Motor neurone disease
   Tumour
   Syringomyelia
   Meningovascular syphilis
   Cord compression (p. 125)
2. *Root lesions*
   Cervical spondylosis
   Neurofibroma, etc.
3. *Brachial plexus lesions*
   Klumpke paralysis
   Cervical rib, etc.
4. *Ulnar or median nerve lesions*
5. *Arthritis of hand or wrist, or disuse atrophy*

Causes of peripheral neuropathy
1. *Idiopathic*
2. *Metabolic*
   Diabetes mellitus
   Amyloidosis
   Acute intermittent porphyria
   Chronic uraemia
   Dysproteinaemia
3. *Vitamin deficiency*
   Subacute combined degeneration (B_{12})
   B complex (alcoholism, beri-beri)
   Pellagra

4. *Infection*
   Diphtheria
   Leprosy
   Tetanus
   Botulism
5. *Drugs and chemicals*
   Isoniazid, nitrofurantoin, vincristine
   Heavy metals (Pb, Hg)
   Organic chemicals, e.g. triorthocresyl phosphate
6. *Miscellaneous*
   Collagen-vascular disease
   Malignancy (Lymphoma or Ca.)
   Sarcoidosis
   Guillain–Barré
   'Brachial neuritis' (neuralgic amyotrophy)
7. *Mechanical*
   Trauma, compression, stretching
8. *Hereditary*
   Hereditary ataxias
   Hereditary sensory radicular neuropathy (Denny–Brown)
   Hypertrophic interstitial neuritis (Déjerine–Sottas)
   Peroneal muscular atrophy (Charcot–Marie–Tooth)
   Refsum's disease

Causes of mononeuritis multiplex
1. Vasculitis, e.g. PN or Wegener's
2. Rheumatoid disease
3. Diabetes mellitus
4. Infection: leprosy, Lyme disease
5. Carcinoma
6. Sarcoidosis
7. Amyloidosis
8. Post-vaccination

Types of non-metastatic carcinomatous neuromyopathy
1. *Encephalopathy*
   (i)   Progressive multifocal leukoencephalopathy
   (ii) Polio-encephalopathy
   (iii) Cerebellar degeneration
   (iv) Dementia
2. *Encephalomyelitis*
3. *Neuropathy*
   Motor, sensory or mixed
4. *Neuromuscular disorder*
   (i)   Myasthenia gravis
   (ii) Eaton Lambert syndrome (weakness which improves with
         tetanic stimulation)
5. *Dermatomyositis or polymyositis*

6. *Non-specific muscle wasting*
7. *Neuromyotonia*
8. *Muscle weakness due to ectopic hormones,* e.g. ACTH or parathormone

Causes of absent knee and ankle jerks with an extensor plantar response (i.e. UMN lesion with dorsal root loss)
1. Subacute combined degeneration
2. Syphilitic tabo-paresis
3. Friedreich's ataxia
4. Motor neurone disease
5. Diabetes mellitus
6. Conus medullaris lesion

ARGYLL ROBERTSON PUPILS

(Accommodation Reflex Present)

The light reflex is interrupted between the lateral geniculate body and the oculomotor nucleus (probably in the pretectal area)

Causes
1. Syphilis, esp. tabes dorsalis
2. Diabetes mellitus
3. Rarely alcoholism, encephalitis, MS or vascular or neoplastic lesions of midbrain

CAUSES OF A CHARCOT JOINT

1. Tabes dorsalis
2. Syringomyelia
3. Diabetes mellitus
Rarely:
4. Cord lesion, e.g. trauma, meningomyelocoele, subacute combined degeneration
5. Leprosy, yaws
6. Congenital neuropathy (p. 129)
7. Congenital indifference to pain
8. Familial dysautonomia (Riley–Day syndrome)
   Includes pain insensitivity due to sensory neuropathy, absent tears, pyrexia, blotchy rash and sweating attacks
9. Repeated intra-articular steroid injection

CAUSES OF TREMOR

1. Parkinsonism
2. Cerebellar lesion
3. Anxiety

4. Thyrotoxicosis
5. Alcoholism
6. Drugs, e.g. tricyclic antidepressants
7. Heavy metals (e.g. 'hatters' shakes' due to mercury)
8. Neurosyphilis
9. Benign essential or familial tremor

CAUSES OF PARKINSONISM

(Tremor, rigidity and hypokinesia)
1. Idiopathic 'paralysis agitans'
2. Drugs—Phenothiazines
           haloperidol
           reserpine
           methyldopa
           tetrabenazine
3. Toxins—manganese
           carbon monoxide
           kernicterus
4. Postencephalitic
5. Repeated head injury
6. Rarely syphilis, cerebral tumour, hypoparathyroidism or Behçet's
Parkinsonian features also occur in
1. Phenylketonuria
2. Hepatolenticular degeneration
3. Shy–Drager syndrome (with postural hypotension due to
   autonomic dysfunction)
4. Progressive supranuclear palsy with paralysis of conjugate gaze
   (Steele–Richardson syndrome)
5. Creutzfeld–Jakob transmissible dementia
6. Olivopontocerebellar atrophy

Atheroma as a cause of parkinsonism is disputed

SIDE-EFFECTS OF NEUROLEPTIC DRUGS

1. *Extrapyramidal*
   Acute dystonia
   Parkinsonism
   Tardive dyskinesia
2. *Autonomic*
   Postural hypotension
   Failure of ejaculation
3. *Anticholinergic*
   Dry mouth, nasal stuffiness, urinary retention, constipation,
   blurred vision, tachycardia

4. *Other CNS effects*
   Mental slowness, headache, nausea, dizziness or paradoxical excitement
5. *Metabolic*
   Weight gain
   Increased serum cholesterol
6. *Rare*
   Cholestasis
   Blood dyscrasias
   Skin pigmentation or rash
   Glaucoma
   Galactorrhoea
   Arrhythmias (prolonged QT, flat T and U waves)
   Pigmentary retinopathy (thioridazine)

CAUSES OF CHOREA

1. Sydenham's chorea—Rheumatic fever
2. Huntington's chorea
3. Drugs   Oral contraceptives
            Neuroleptics
            Phenytoin
4. Pregnancy
5. Thyrotoxicosis
6. Polycythaemia
7. SLE
8. Senile chorea
9. CO poisoning

CAUSES OF DISORDERED NEUROMUSCULAR TRANSMISSION

1. *Hereditary*
   (i)   Hereditary myasthenia gravis
   (ii)   Pseudocholinesterase deficiency (suxamethonium paralysis)
2. *Drugs and toxins*
   (i)   Depolarizing drugs
   (ii)   Anticholinesterase poisons (e.g. 'nerve gas')
   (iii)   Botulism
   (iv)   Venom of Black Widow spider, puff-fish, etc.
   (v)   Magnesium poisoning
   (vi)   Antibiotics, especially kanamycin
3. *Idiopathic myasthenia gravis*
   (possibly autoimmune)
4. *Myasthenia associated with other disease*
   (i)   Thyrotoxicosis
   (ii)   Malignancy (Eaton Lambert syndrome)
   (iii)   SLE or polymyositis

MYOTONIA

1. *Myotonia congenita*
   Thomson: Dominant
   Becker: Recessive, more severe and later onset
2. *Dystrophia myotonica*
   (i)   Myotonia and muscle atrophy
   (ii) Characteristic facies with ptosis and frontal baldness
   (iii) Cataracts, gonadal atrophy, heart disease, hypoventilation,
         bone changes and dementia
3. *Paramyotonia congenita*
   Myotonia and weakness induced by cold, sometimes with
   fluctuation in serum potassium

PROGRESSIVE MUSCULAR DYSTROPHIES

1. *X linked recessive ('Pseudo-hypertrophic')*
   (i) Duchenne (severe)
   (ii) Becker (milder and of later onset)
2. *Autosomal recessive*
   Limb girdle type (Erb)
3. *Autosomal dominant*
   (i)   Facio-scapulo-humeral (Landouzy and Déjerine)
   (ii) Distal myopathy of late onset (Welander)
   (iii) Ocular myopathy (may also be either retinopathy or
         dysphagia)
Certain exceptions occur to this simple genetic classification

METABOLIC AND ENDOCRINE MYOPATHIES

1. *Periodic paralysis*
   Serum K may fall, rise or remain constant during attacks
2. *Glycogen storage diseases*
3. *Mitochondrial overactivity*
   (i) Hypermetabolic myopathy
   (ii) Malignant hyperpyrexia during anaesthesia
4. *Nutritional myopathy*
   (i) Kwashiorkor
   (ii) Vitamin E deficiency
5. *Drugs*
   (i)   Glucocorticoids, especially triamcinolone
   (ii) Alcohol
   (iii) Drugs which induce hypokalaemia
   (iv) Heroin, amphetamine addiction
   (v)   Chloroquine
   (vi) Vincristine

6. *Endocrine*
    (i)   Hyper- or hypothyroidism
    (ii) Osteomalacia
    (iii) Acromegaly
    (iv) Cushing's syndrome
    (v)   Hypoadrenalism
    (vi) Primary aldosteronism

IMPORTANT CAUSES OF PROXIMAL MYOPATHY

1. Hereditary limb girdle myopathy
2. Polymyositis/dermatomyositis
3. Carcinomatous myopathy
4. Metabolic or endocrine
    (i)   Cushing's or glucocorticoid therapy
    (ii) Thyrotoxicosis
    (iii) Osteomalacia
5. Polymyalgia rheumatica
6. Idiopathic (esp. elderly females)

Terms which are sometimes confused

1. *Dysphasia.* Cortical disorder in use of symbols for
   communication, whether spoken, heard, written or read
   Dysarthria. Disorder of articulation of speech

2. *Apraxia.* Inability to carry out purposive learned movements in
   absence of motor paralysis, sensory loss or ataxia
   Agnosia. Failure to recognize, whether visual, auditory or tactile

3. *Perseveration.* Continuation or recurrence of an activity without
   appropriate stimulus
   Verbigeration. Meaningless repetition of words or sentences
   Echolalia. Parrot-like repetition by the subject of statements or
   acts made before them

4. *Epilepsy.* A paroxysmal transitory disturbance of brain function,
   ceasing spontaneously, with a tendency to recurrence
   Myoclonus. A brief shock-like contraction of a number of
   muscle fibres, a whole muscle or several muscles, either
   simultaneously or successively

5. *Fibrillation.* Spontaneous contraction of individual muscle fibres
   (EMG finding)
   Fasciculation. Spontaneous contraction of bundles of fibres in
   the same motor unit (seen clinically)

6. *Amaurosis.* Blindness from any cause
   Amblyopia. Poor vision not due to retractive error or ocular disease

7. *Athetosis.* Involuntary slow coarse writhing movements, usually most pronounced in hand or arms
   Dystonia. Involuntary sustained twisting movements, usually affecting proximal muscles

Endocrine and bone disease

THE HYPOTHALAMUS

FUNCTIONS OF HYPOTHALAMUS

1. **CNS control centres**
   - (i) Sleep
   - (ii) Temperature
   - (iii) Thirst
   - (iv) Appetite
   - (v) Memory
   - (vi) Autonomic activity

2. **Direct hormone secretion** (via axonal transport to posterior pituitary)
   - (i) Oxytocin
   - (ii) Vasopression
   - (iii) Neurophysin

3. **Releasing hormones** (via portal capillaries)
Control of anterior pituitary

HYPOTHALAMIC REGULATORY HORMONES

Thyrotrophin releasing hormone—TRH
Releases
   - (i) TSH and prolactin in both sexes
   - (ii) FSH in men
   - (iii) GH in some patients with acromegaly and renal failure

Luteinizing/follicle-stimulating hormone releasing factor—LH/FSH-RH
Releases
   - (i) LH and FSH in both sexes
   - (ii) GH in some patients with acromegaly

Somatostatin—GH-RIH
Somatostatin is found in the hypothalamus, pancreatic islet cells, gut and elsewhere. It is secreted by some endocrine tumours

(somatostatinomas), e.g. small cell Ca lung, medullary Ca thyroid
Suppresses
  (i)   GH in normal subjects and acromegalic patients
  (ii) Many regulatory peptides ('endocrine cyanide')
  (iii) Insulin, glucagon and gastrin release

CAUSES OF HYPOTHALAMIC DYSFUNCTION

1. Development defect, e.g. chronic hydrocephalus
2. Tumours of CNS, including metastases
3. Granuloma, e.g. sarcoid, TB
4. Infection, e.g. encephalitis
5. Vascular, e.g. infarction, subarachnoid haemorrhage
6. Degenerative disease, e.g. Wernicke's
7. Trauma, surgery or cranial irradiation
8. Stress, e.g. emotional deprivation in children
9. Drugs, e.g. dopamine antagonists

ANTERIOR PITUITARY HORMONES

1. Adrenocorticortrophic hormone (ACTH)
Pro-opiomelanocortin is the precursor molecule:

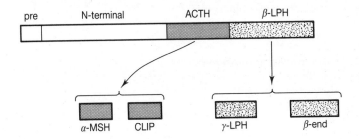

Endogenous opiates
These peptides (endorphins and enkephalins) which are derived
from the β-lipotrophin portion of the ACTH precursor molecule have
similar actions to morphine and may regulate basal neural
transmission. They occur in the CNS, sympathetic ganglia, adrenal
medulla, gastrointestinal tract and pancreas

2. Growth hormone (GH)
Controlled by two hypothalamic polypeptides:
  1. GRF (growth hormone releasing factor) stimulates GH
  2. Somatostatin suppresses GH
GH acts via *somatomedin* to increase circulating free fatty acids,
blood sugar and protein synthesis

Insulin-like growth factors, IGF-1 and -2 (somatomedins), show a molecular resemblance to the A and B chains of insulin. The cell surface receptors for IGF are similar to the insulin receptors. IGF -1 is *increased* in acromegaly, and *decreased* in GH deficiency, malnutrition, hepatic or renal failure and uncontrolled diabetes. IGF -1 controls GH secretion by negative feedback inhibition. IGF inhibitors occur in insulin deficiency and may explain the increased GH seen in uncontrolled diabetes

3. Thyroid stimulating hormone (TSH)

Stimulated by	*Suppressed by*
TRH	Dopamine
	Somatostatin
	Thyroxine

4. Prolactin (PRL)

Stimulated by	*Suppressed by*
Stress	Hypothalamic prolactin
Suckling	inhibitor
Oestrogens	Dopaminergic drugs
TRH	Bromocryptine
Serotonin	
Hypoglycaemia	
Drugs—dopaminergic blockers	
morphine	
methyldopa	

5. Follicle-stimulating hormone (FSH)

Stimulated by	*Suppressed by*
Gonadotrophin-releasing	Oestrogen
hormone (GnRH)	Progestogen
Clomiphene	Androgen
	Inhibin

6. Luteinizing hormone (LH)

Stimulated by	*Suppressed by*
Gonadotrophin-releasing	Oestrogen
hormone (GnRH)	Progestogen
Clomiphene	Androgen

CAUSES OF HYPOPITUITARISM

1. *Congenital*
   Solitary GH deficiency or combined, e.g. LH, TSH, Kallman's syndrome
2. *Tumours*
   (i) Eosinophil adenoma
   (ii) Chromophobe adenoma

    (iii) Craniopharyngioma
    (iv) Metastatic cancer
3. *Iatrogenic*
   Hypophysectomy or irradiation
4. *Vascular*
   Pituitary apoplexy, Sheehan's syndrome
5. *Infection*
   Meningitis, tuberculosis
6. *Trauma*
   Fracture of base of skull
7. *Infiltration*
   Sarcoid, Langerhans cell histiocytosis
8. *Others*
   Anorexia nervosa
   Malnutrition

POSTERIOR PITUITARY HORMONES

1. Oxytocin

Stimulated by	*Suppressed by*
Acetylcholine	Catecholamine (β-effect)
Angiotensin II	Stress
Sexual intercourse	
Parturition	
Suckling	

2. Vasopressin (arginine-vasopressin, antidiuretic hormone, ADH)
Controlled by:
    (i) *Plasma osmolality.* ADH secretion increases as osmolality
       rises
    (ii) *Extracellular fluid volume.* Stretch receptors in thorax and
       left atrium detect changes in plasma volume.
       10% depletion of plasma volume increases ADH secretion

CAUSES OF DIABETES INSIPIDUS

A. Neurogenic

Primary	Idiopathic
	Familial
	DIDMOAD syndrome (see p. 145)
Secondary	Infection—Meningitis, abscess, TB
	Tumours—primary or secondary
	Infiltration—Sarcoidosis
	Iatrogenic—Surgery or radiotherapy
	Vascular—Sheehan's, CVA
	Trauma

B. Nephrogenic

Genetic	X-linked
Metabolic	Hypokalaemia
	Hypercalcaemia
Drugs	Lithium carbonate, demeclocycline,
	amphotericin B, glibenclamide, gentamycin

CAUSES OF GYNAECOMASTIA

1. Hermaphroditism or pseudo-hermaphroditism (p. 143)
2. Endocrine
   Normal puberty and neonatal
   Hypothyroidism
   Thyrotoxicosis
   Hypoadrenalism
   Hyperparathyroidism
   Testicular atrophy
   Testicular and adrenal tumours
   Acromegaly
   Hypothalamic lesions
3. Cirrhosis
4. Carcinoma or lymphoma
5. Refeeding after malnutrition
6. Renal failure with dialysis
7. Paraplegia
8. Erythroderma
9. Leprosy
10. Drugs
    Sex hormones (both androgens and oestrogens)
    Antiandrogens
       Cyproterone acetate
       Flutamide
       Spironolactone
       Ketoconazole
       Cimetidine
    Amphetamine
    Reserpine
    Digitalis
    Methyldopa

CAUSES OF GALACTORRHOEA

1. Physiological (post-partum and neonatal)
2. Prolonged stress
3. Prolactin-secreting pituitary tumour
4. Pituitary stalk or hypothalamic lesion
5. Ectopic prolactin production, e.g. bronchial Ca.

6. Drugs, e.g.
   Phenothiazines
   Oral contraceptives
   Opiates
   Haloperidol
   Tricyclic antidepressants
   Methyldopa
   Meprobamate
   Reserpine
7. Chest wall injury (surgery, herpes zoster, mesothelioma)
   Probably stimulates neurological pathway of suckling reflex
8. Hysterectomy
9. Polycystic ovary syndrome
10. Hypothyroidism

CAUSES OF AMENORRHOEA

Physiological
   1. Prepubertal
   2. Pregnancy
   3. Menopausal

Pathological
   1. *Anatomical*
      (i)   Uterine anomaly
      (ii) Hysterectomy
      (iii) Cryptomenorrhoea
   2. *Hypothalamic-pituitary axis*
      (i)   'Functional' amenorrhoea: change in environment, emotional upset, rapid change in weight (esp. anorexia nervosa)
      (ii)   Severe systemic disease: e.g. TB
      (iii) Hyperprolactinaemia
      (iv)   Hypopituitarism
      (v)   Isolated gonadotrophin deficiency
      (vi)   Thyrotoxicosis
      (vii) Drugs: oestrogen, progesterone, testosterone, glucocorticoids, spironolactone
   3. *Primary ovarian disease*
      (i)   Oophorectomy
      (ii) Irradiation or cytotoxic drugs
      (iii) Pelvic TB
      (iv) Autoimmune, e.g. associated with Addison's disease
   4. *Virilizing syndromes*
      (i) Genetic intersex (p. 143)
      (ii) Ovarian
           Stein–Leventhal syndrome (polycystic ovary)
           Virilizing tumours, e.g. androblastoma

(iii)   Adrenal
Congenital adrenal hyperplasia
Acquired virilizing adenoma or Ca.
5. *Oestrogen or progesterone excess*
  (i)   Follicular or lutein retention cyst
 (ii)   Sex cord stromal tumours

ORAL CONTRACEPTIVES

Long term effects

Definitely protect against:
1. Menstrual irregularity
2. Iron deficiency anaemia
3. Benign breast disease
4. Functional ovarian cysts
5. Ovarian cancer
6. Endometrial cancer

May protect against:
1. Thyroid disorders
2. Rheumatoid arthritis
3. Peptic ulcer
4. Pelvic inflammatory disease

Definitely predispose to:
1. Hypertension
2. Venous thromboembolism
3. Thrombotic stroke
4. Haemorrhagic stroke
5. Hepatocellular adenoma
6. Impaired fertility (temporary, after stopping)
7. Chloasma, spider naevi

May predispose to:
1. Cancer of cervix, breast, liver or malignant melanoma (in some subgroups or long-term users)
2. Gall-bladder disease
3. Inflammatory bowel disease
4. Migraine
5. Depression
6. Urinary tract infection
7. Fetal malformation if taken during pregnancy

FEMALE HYPOGONADISM

Clinical features may include failure of puberty, primary or secondary amenorrhoea, infertility and early menopause

1. **Low gonadotrophin**
   (i)   Hypothalamic disorder, e.g. stress, anorexia nervosa or Kallman's syndrome (GnRH deficiency)
  (ii)   Pituitary tumour, infarct, granuloma, etc.
 (iii)   Ovarian or adrenal disorder, e.g. androgen- or oestrogen-secreting tumours or congenital adrenal hyperplasia with virilization

2. **Raised gonadotrophin**
   (i)   Ovarian failure, e.g. agenesis, dysgenesis, polycystic ovary syndrome, radiotherapy, etc.

3. **Genetic intersexual states**
   e.g. Turner's (XO) (see below)

CAUSES OF PRECOCIOUS PUBERTY

A. **True precocity** (premature activation of pituitary-hypothalamic axis)
   1. *Constitutional* (usually female, may be familial)
   2. *Secondary*
      (i) Tumours near the hypothalamus, e.g. pinealoma, hamartoma, teratoma, etc.
      (ii) Brain damage, e.g. encephalitis, hydrocephalus, etc.
      (iii) Polyostotic fibrous dysplasia (Albright's syndrome)
      (iv) Hepatic cell carcinoma

B. **Pseudo-precocity** (secondary sexual development with immature gonads)
Overproduction of androgen or oestrogen by
   (i) Disease of ovary, testis or adrenal
   (ii) Teratoma
   (iii) Exogenous hormone

INTERSEXUAL STATES

True hermaphrodites have both testicular and ovarian elements in the gonads
Male pseudo-hermaphrodites have testes but are feminized
Female pseudo-hermaphrodites have ovaries but are virilized

Causes
   1. *Genetic*
      (i) Turner's: XO
      (ii) Chromatin positive ovarian dysgenesis
          Abnormal X
          Mosaics
      (iii) Klinefelter's: XXY
      (iv) Mosaics: XY/XO, XX/XY, etc.
      (v) Gonadal dysgenesis: female phenotype
   2. *Hormonal*
      Female
      (i) Congenital adrenal hyperplasia
      (ii) Virilizing tumour of mother during pregnancy
      (iii) Sex hormones given to mother during pregnancy, e.g. to prevent abortion
      Male
      (i) End-organ unresponsiveness to androgens (testicular feminization)
      (ii) Deficiency of 5α-reductase, which converts T to dihydro-T

CAUSES OF SHORT STATURE

1. **'Constitutional'**
   Racial, familial or sporadic

2. **Nutritional**
   (i)   Starvation
   (ii) Malabsorption
   (iii) Protein loss

3. **Chromosomal defects**
   (i) Trisomies, e.g. Down's
   (ii) Turner's

4. **Skeletal defects**
   (i)   Rickets
   (ii) Achondroplasia
   (iii) Gargoylism (Hurler's)

5. **Chronic systemic disease**
   (i)   Cyanotic congenital heart disease
   (ii)   Renal failure
   (iii) Hepatic failure
   (iv)   Pulmonary disease
   (v)   Anaemia
   (vi)   Infections, e.g. TB
   (vii) Long-term steroid therapy (e.g. for asthma)

6. **Endocrine disease**
   (i)   Sexual precocity
   (ii) Hypopituitarism
   (iii) Hypothyroidism
   (iv) Congenital adrenal hyperplasia

7. **Miscellaneous rare diseases**
   Diseases of unknown cause, e.g. progeria

DIABETES MELLITUS

Definition: Diabetes mellitus is a syndrome which merges with the normal, and diagnostic criteria are therefore arbitrary. The British Diabetic Association has adopted the 1980 WHO recommendations:
   1. If diabetic symptoms are present, a random venous plasma glucose value of 11 mmol/l or more, or a fasting value of 8 mmol/l or more, is diagnostic of diabetes. Postprandial values below 8 mmol/l and fasting values below 6 mmol/l exclude the diagnosis
   2. If these results are equivocal, an oral glucose tolerance test (using 75 g glucose) is performed. In 'impaired glucose

tolerance' the fasting venous plasma value is less than
8 mmol/l, but 2 hours after the glucose load the value is
between 8 and 11 mmol/l (For whole venous blood, the values
are 1 mmol/l lower)
Plasma C-peptide levels after glucagon stimulation may be used
to distinguish insulin-dependent from insulin-independent
patients, the levels being higher in the latter (> 1.8 ng/ml)

Causes of diabetes mellitus
1. *Idiopathic*
   - (i)   Subclinical—Impaired glucose tolerance
   - (ii) Clinical—Insulin-dependent ('juvenile onset')
             Non-insulin-dependent ('maturity onset')
2. *Secondary to other disease*
   - (i)   Pancreatic disease (pancreatitis, Ca., haemochromatosis, etc.)
   - (ii) Peripheral antagonism to insulin
     - a. Glucocorticoids, e.g. Cushing's
     - b. Glucagonoma
     - c. Acromegaly
   - (iii) Insulin receptor defects
     - a. Congenital lipodystrophy
     - b. With acanthosis nigricans
   - (iv) Hypoinsulinaemia
     - a. Phaeochromocytoma
     - b. Somatostatinoma
     - c. Hyperaldosteronism
   - (v)   Cirrhosis
3. *Drugs*
   - (i)   Glucocorticoids
   - (ii) Oral contraceptives
   - (iii) Thiazides
   - (iv) Diazoxide
   - (v)   Pancreatic toxins, e.g. cytotoxics, alloxan
4. *Genetic syndromes*
   - (i)   Glycogen storage type 1
   - (ii) DIDMOAD (diabetes insipidus, DM, optic atrophy and deafness)
   - (iii) Laurence–Moon–Biedl syndrome
   - (iv) Down's syndrome

Chronic complications of diabetes mellitus
1. *Ocular*
   - (i)   Blurred vision due to fluctuations in blood sugar
   - (ii) Cataracts
   - (iii) Retinopathy:
             Venous engorgement
             Capillary microaneurysms

'Blot' haemorrhages
'Waxy' exudates
Retinal infarcts ('cottonwool spots')
Vitreous haemorrhage
Retinitis proliferans
Retinal detachment
  (iv) Rubeosis iridis (new blood vessels over iris)—may cause
        glaucoma
2. *Neurological*
   (i) Cerebral disturbance due to hyper- or hypo-glycaemia
  (ii) Cerebral lesions due to atheroma
 (iii) Peripheral neuropathy
        a. Asymptomatic loss of ankle-jerks and vibration sense
        b. Painful subacute neuritis, usually in lower limbs
        c. Mononeuritis multiplex (often asymmetrical)
        d. Isolated cranial nerve lesions
        e. Autonomic neuropathy
  (iv) Diabetic pseudotabes
   (v) Diabetic amyotrophy
  (vi) 'Insulin neuritis' during stabilization
3. *Renal*
   (i) Pyelonephritis, sometimes with papillary necrosis
  (ii) Glomerulonephritis
        a. Kimmelstiel–Wilson (eosinophilic nodules in glomerular
           tuft)
        b. Proliferative, with sclerosed basement membrane
 (iii) Atherosclerosis and hypertensive vascular changes
4. *Vascular*
   Occlusion of large vessels (atheroma) or small vessels
   (endarteritis) may cause ischaemia of feet, myocardium, brain
   or kidneys
5. *Dermatological*
   (i) Fat atrophy or hypertrophy or fibrosis at insulin injection
        sites
  (ii) Ulcers due to neuropathy or ischaemia
 (iii) Infections, especially furuncles and Candidosis
  (iv) Pigmented scars over shins ('diabetic dermopathy')
   (v) Xanthomata
  (vi) Necrobiosis lipoidica
 (vii) Widespread granuloma annulare
6. *Systemic infections*
   Incidence of TB, chronic urinary infections and deep mycoses is
   increased
7. *Psychological and social*

Glycosylated haemoglobin
Correlates with the degree of hyperglycaemia in the preceding 6
weeks *(contd)*

Causes of false increase
1. Presence of HbF, e.g. pregnancy, thalassaemia
2. Carbamylated haemoglobin, e.g. uraemia

Causes of false decrease
1. Haemolytic anaemia
2. HbS or HbC

DIABETES AND PREGNANCY

Pregnancy produces a tendency to both ketoacidosis and fasting hypoglycaemia. This paradox is due to
1. Counteraction of maternal insulin by placental hormones
2. Removal of glucose by the fetus

COMPLICATIONS OF PREGNANCY IN THE DIABETIC

1. *Maternal morbidity*
   (i) Hydramnios
   (ii) Pre-eclampsia
   (iii) Pregnancy probably accelerates diabetic microangiopathy and some authors recommend abortion and sterilization in women with proliferative retinopathy or nephropathy
2. *Fetal mortality.* Still-birth (5–10%) or neonatal death (5–10%) due to
   (i) Hyaline membrane disease (preterm delivery)
   (ii) Congenital anomalies (often cardiac or neurological)
3. *Fetal morbidity*
   (i) Macrosomia (excessive size)
   (ii) Hypoglycaemia
   (iii) Congenital anomalies
   (iv) Respiratory distress (due to preterm delivery)
   (v) Hypocalcaemia (maternal hypercalcaemia suppresses the fetal parathyroid)

CAUSES OF HYPOGLYCAEMIA

1. *Starvation and exercise*
2. *Reaction to glucose ingestion*
   Functional
   Early diabetes mellitus
   Postgastrectomy
3. *β-cell overactivity*
   Insulinoma
   Hyperplasia
4. *Endocrine disease*
   Hypothyroidism
   Hypopituitarism
   Hypoadrenalism

5. *Drugs*
   Insulin
   Oral hypoglycaemics
   Salicylates
   Paracetamol
   Ackee, etc.
6. *Sensitivity to:*
   Leucine
   Galactose, fructose
   Alcohol, tobacco
7. *Liver disease*
   Glycogen storage disease
   Hepatoma
8. *Neoplasm*
   Especially large fibrosarcoma
9. *In infancy*
   (i) Idiopathic hypoglycaemia of infancy
   (ii) After fetal malnutrition

LIPOPROTEIN METABOLISM

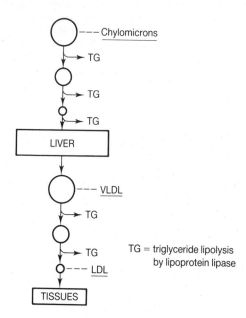

TG = triglyceride lipolysis
by lipoprotein lipase

Chylomicrons are large lipoprotein particles which enter the blood from the lymphatics via the thoracic duct. Lipoprotein lipase which is attached to the vascular endothelium then causes serial lipolysis to form progressively smaller but denser chylomicron remnants (high density lipoproteins), which enter the liver

The liver then synthesizes and excretes into the blood *very low density lipoproteins* (VLDL) which are similarly broken down to form the *low density lipoproteins* (LDL) which are rich in cholesterol. LDL then delivers the cholesterol to the cells of the tissues where it is needed for membrane growth and steroidogenesis

LDL uptake into the cells is controlled by receptors, and the synthesis of these receptors is suppressed when the cell does not require further cholesterol. With low levels of LDL this mechanism controls the cell's uptake of LDL, but with high blood levels of LDL the LDL also enters the cells by a non-receptor route

High density lipoproteins (HDL) in the blood take up cholesterol for excretion into the bile via the liver

Thus increased LDL predispose to atheroma, and HDL protect against atheroma

Scavenger macrophages in the blood can take up excess LDL and become converted to foam cells

Electrophoretic strip

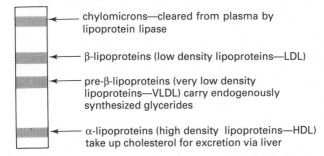

chylomicrons—cleared from plasma by lipoprotein lipase

β-lipoproteins (low density lipoproteins—LDL)

pre-β-lipoproteins (very low density lipoproteins—VLDL) carry endogenously synthesized glycerides

α-lipoproteins (high density lipoproteins—HDL) take up cholesterol for excretion via liver

Tangier disease
HDL is defective and cholesterol accumulates in reticuloendothelial tissues

Primary hyperlipoproteinaemia (WHO classification)
This is not a diagnostic classification. It simply reports which lipid levels are raised, and a patient's type may change during treatment

Type	Lipoprotein increase
I	Chylomicrons
II a	LDL
II b	LDL & VLDL

III	Floating beta (broad beta, remnants)
IV	VLDL
V	Chylomicrons and VLDL

Secondary hyperlipoproteinaemia

Causes
1. Diabetes mellitus
2. Hypothyroidism
3. Chronic renal failure or nephrotic syndrome
4. Cholestasis (especially primary biliary cirrhosis)
5. Pancreatitis
6. Drugs—Retinoids
        Beta-blockers
        Oestrogen
        Corticosteroids
        Thiazides
7. Alcoholism
8. Obesity
9. Pregnancy

Conditions associated with severe hyperlipoproteinaemia
1. Ischaemic heart disease
2. Peripheral atheroma
3. Xanthoma
4. Pancreatitis
5. Lipaemia retinalis
6. Hepatosplenomegaly
7. Gout
8. Tendinitis
9. Aortic stenosis

Clinical types of xanthomas
1. Plane   —in palm creases and eyelid (xanthelasma)
2. Tendon   —nodules attached to tendons or ligaments
3. Tuberous   —larger lesions which may be tender
4. Eruptive   —multiple small lesions occurring in 'showers', often
               with a red halo

Palmar crease xanthoma suggests either cholestasis or Type 3
Xanthelasma suggests Type 2, but can occur in normal people

CONGENITAL ADRENAL HYPERPLASIA

Cortisol, aldosterone and androgen synthesis may be affected depending on site of enzyme block

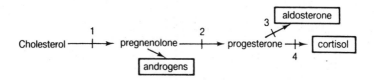

Site 1
Lipoid hyperplasia (20–22 desmolase deficiency). Very rare
Severe deficiency in all 3 hormones

Site 2
3β-hydroxysteroid dehydrogenase defect. Very rare
Androgens unaffected

Site 3
21β-hydroxylase defect
Clinical features
   (i)   Ambiguous genitalia
   (ii) Virilization in female, precocious pseudo-puberty in male
   (iii) Electrolyte imbalance
   (iv) Rapid growth, but eventual short stature
The plasma 17-hydroxyprogesterone is increased

Site 4
11β-hydroxylase defect
Hypertension with virilization

CAUSES OF ADRENAL INSUFFICIENCY

Primary
   1. Acute or chronic gland destruction
      (i)   Autoimmune adrenalitis
      (ii) Infection: TB, fungal (esp. histoplasmosis)
      (iii) Infiltration: metastasis, amyloidosis, haemochromatosis
      (iv) Haemorrhage (especially meningococcal septicaemia, or in neonate after breech delivery)
      (v)   Adrenalectomy (bilateral)
      (vi) Adrenal vein thrombosis (e.g. after adrenal venography)
   2. Metabolic failure
      (i)   Virilizing hyperplasia, e.g. C21-hydroxylase deficiency
      (ii) Enzyme inhibitors, e.g. metyrapone

   (iii) Cytotoxic drugs, e.g. opDDD
   (iv) Other drugs: etomidate, ketoconazole
    (v) Adrenoleukodystrophy
   (vi) Congenital adrenal hypoplasia

Secondary
  1. Hypopituitarism
  2. Suppression of hypothalamic-pituitary axis
     (i) Exogenous glucocorticoids
    (ii) Endogenous glucocorticoids, e.g. Cushing's syndrome
          following tumour removal

RENIN, ANGIOTENSIN AND ALDOSTERONE

Substrate globulin (angiotensinogen)
in blood

Renin release (from juxta-glomerular apparatus)

Angiotensin I

Converting enzyme

Inhibits

B.P. increase

Extracellular fluid volume increase

Sodium retention

Angiotensin II and III

Stimulates

Aldosterone secretion (from adrenal)

Angiotensinase

Inactive forms

Angiotensin II also has a pressor effect by direct vasoconstriction
Saralasin competitively antagonizes the acute pressor effect of
angiotensin II
Captopril and enalapril inhibit the enzyme that converts angiotensin
I to angiotensin II

Atrial natriuretic peptides

A series of peptides secreted by granules in the atria of the heart have been shown to decrease sodium and water retention. They are released by a rise in atrial pressure and probably help to control blood pressure

Actions
1. Decrease salt and water retention by the kidney
2. Relax smooth muscle in vessels, especially in the renal vessels
3. Inhibit release of aldosterone, especially that provoked by angiotensin II

The juxtaglomerular apparatus

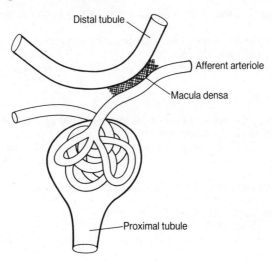

Aldosterone

Stimulated by loss of sodium
                retention of potassium
                fall in extracellular fluid volume
Inhibited by atrial natriuretic hormone

Causes of hyperaldosteronism

Primary (rare)
1. Conn's tumour (adrenal adenoma)
2. Adrenal hyperplasia or carcinoma

Secondary
1. Hypertension
2. Diuretic therapy
3. Fluid retention (nephrotic syndrome, cirrhosis, cardiac failure)

4. Renal:
   (i)   Salt-losing nephropathy
   (ii)   Tubular acidosis
   (iii) Renal tumour
   (iv)   Bartter's syndrome (with hyperplasia of the
          juxtaglomerular apparatus, resistance to the pressor
          effects of angiotensin II, and overproduction of
          prostaglandins)
   (v)   Renin hypersecretion

Regulators of renin release
1. Receptors in the afferent arterioles are sensitive to the
   perfusion pressure
2. Receptors in the macula densa are sensitive to the sodium
   levels
3. Circulating hormones (e.g. vasopressin, angiotensin I and II)
   can inhibit renin release
4. Sympathetic nerve stimulation increases renin release

THE THYROID

The thyroid secretes T3 (5 nmol/day) and T4 (100 nmol/day). More
than 99% of each is protein-bound
   T4 (active) is converted to T3 (active) and reverse T3 (inactive) in
the peripheral tissues, and T3 has thrice the metabolic activity of T4

Impaired conversion of T4 to T3 occurs in:
1. Fetus, infant and elderly
2. Malignancy or starvation
3. Hepatic or renal disease
4. Drugs, e.g. amiodarone, propranolol, propythiouracil and
   dexamethasone

CAUSES OF HYPOTHYROIDISM

A. Primary (thyroid gland failure)
   1. Congenital
      (i)   Absence of maldevelopment of thyroid gland
      (ii)   Endemic cretinism (maternal iodine deficiency)
      (iii) Dyshormonogenesis (enzyme defects affect hormone
             synthesis)
             e.g. peroxidase deficiency
   2. Autoimmune thyroiditis
   3. Iatrogenic
      (i)   Surgery
      (ii)   Irradiation
      (iii) Antithyroid drugs
      (iv)   Goitrogens (lithium, phenylbutazone, PAS)

4. Dietary iodine deficiency
5. Acquired enzyme defects due to dietary goitrogens
6. Riedel's thyroiditis (very rare)

B. Secondary (TSH deficiency)
1. Hypopituitarism
2. Rarely hypothalamic lesion (TRH deficiency)

CAUSES OF HYPERTHYROIDISM

1. Graves' disease and toxic multinodular goitre ⎫ more than
2. Toxic adenoma ⎭ 95% of cases
3. Iatrogenic
    (i) Overdosage with thyroid hormone
    (ii) Following administration of iodine to goitrous patient
        (Jod–Basedow phenomenon)
    (iii) Amiodarone
4. Transient, associated with thyroiditis
5. Ectopic TSH secretion by neoplasm, e.g. choriocarcinoma
6. Ectopic thyroid secretion by struma ovarii
7. Metastatic thyroid cancer
8. Excessive TRH or TSH secretion
9. Polyostotic fibrous dysplasia

T3-TOXICOSIS

Raised serum T3 with normal T4 and flat TSH response on TRH
test. Occurs in about 5% of thyrotoxic patients

Causes
1. Early phase of diffuse goitre toxicity
2. Hot nodule
3. T3 ingestion

CAUSES OF PROPTOSIS

1. *Dysthyroid exophthalmos,* usually with lid retraction, lid lag
   and weak upward gaze
   CAT scan shows enlarged extraocular muscles, and TRH test
   shows abnormal TSH response
2. *Neoplasm*
    (i) Benign, e.g. dermoid
    (ii) Malignant, primary or secondary
3. *Vascular*, e.g. capillary haemangioma
4. *Bony malformation*
5. *Inflammation*, e.g. pseudotumour, orbital cellulitis
6. *Systemic disease*, e.g. Wegener's, histiocytosis X (Langerhans),
   xanthogranuloma, sarcoidosis

THYROID HORMONE BINDING GLOBULIN (TBG)

Causes of increased TBG
1. Pregnancy, oestrogen therapy
2. Drugs, e.g. clofibrate, phenothiazines
3. Viral hepatitis and chronic liver disease
4. Myxoedema

Causes of decreased TBG
1. Hypoproteinaemia (e.g. nephrotic syndrome)
2. Acromegaly
3. Glucocorticoids, androgens and anabolic steroids
4. Malnutrition or major illness
5. Thyrotoxicosis

Causes of reduced TBG binding
1. Renal failure
2. Salicylates, phenytoin, phenylbutazone

MULTIPLE ENDOCRINE NEOPLASIA SYNDROMES

Type I (Werner)
Variable degrees of hyperplasia, adenoma or cancer of pituitary, parathyroid and pancreas

Type IIa (Sipple)
Medullary carcinoma of thyroid, phaeochromocytoma and hyperparathyroidism

Type IIb
Medullary carcinoma of thyroid, phaeochromocytoma and mucosal neuromas, often with pigmentation and Marfanoid habitus

Type IIIa
Phaeochromocytoma, duodenal carcinoid and neurofibromatosis

Type IIIb
Phaeochromocytoma, islet cell tumour and von Hippel–Lindau syndrome

Polyendocrine deficiency syndromes

Type I
Hypoparathyroidism, hypoadrenalism and mucocutaneous candidiasis. Alopecia, pernicious anaemia, malabsorption and chronic active hepatitis also occur

Type II (Schmidt)
Hypoadrenalism, autoimmune thyroid disease and insulin-
dependent diabetes mellitus
Both types I and II can be associated with vitiligo and gonadal
failure

Ectopic humoral syndromes
1. *ACTH and related peptides* (esp. oat cell Ca.)
   May account for 20% of cases of Cushing's syndrome
   Suspect the diagnosis in any patient with:
   (i)   tumour + hypokalaemia
   (ii) Cushing's + high ACTH and cortisol
   (iii) Cushing's + hypokalaemia
   Confirm the diagnosis by:
   (i)   Plasma ACTH: high
   (ii) 24 hr metapyrone test: usually no rise in ACTH in
         response to falling cortisol
   (iii) High dose dexamethasone text: usually no suppression
   (iv) ACTH measurement during selective venous catheterization
   (v)   CAT scan may help, e.g. for thymic tumour
2. *Malignant hypercalcaemia* (esp. breast and lung Ca.)
   Possible mediators include:
   (i)   Ectopic parathormone (rare)
   (ii) Prostaglandins
   (iii) Osteoclast-activating factor
   (iv) Vitamin D-like steroids
3. *Vasopressin* (esp. oat cell Ca.)
   Causes inappropriate diuresis
4. *Gonadotrophin* (esp. in tumours of testis, liver, stomach or
   pancreas)
   Causes precocious puberty in boys, and gynaecomastia in adult
   males
5. *Calcitonin* (esp. oat cell Ca.)
   Occurs in about 50% of lung Ca. patients, but most are
   normocalcaemic
6. *Growth hormone or prolactin*
   Carcinoid may secrete GH-releasing factor
7. *Human placental lactogen*
   Causes gynaecomastia in males
8. *Thyrotrophin* (esp. in trophoblastic neoplasia, e.g. hydatidiform
   mole)
9. *Gastrointestinal hormones* (esp. VIP and somatostatin)
10. *Serotin or catecholamines* (carcinoid and phaeochromocytoma)
11. *Pigmentation* (hormone unknown)
12. *Red cell aplasia or polycythaemia* (erythropoietin)
13. *Prostaglandin E_2*
14. *Insulin*
    Doubtful entity, and hypoglycaemia may have other causes

VITAMIN D SYNTHESIS

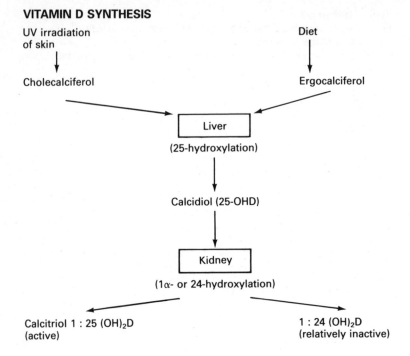

CALCIUM HOMEOSTASIS

Blood calcium is regulated by 3 hormones

1. Parathyroid hormone (PTH)
A fall in blood calcium ions increases PTH secretion

Actions of PTH
  (i)   Directly inhibits resorption of phosphate in the renal
        proximal tubule
  (ii) Promotes reabsorption of calcium in the distal tubule
  (iii) Stimulates 1 : 25 dihydroxyvitamin D formation in the kidney
  (iv) Acts via the osteoclasts to liberate calcium from bone

2. 1 : 25 dihydroxyvitamin D (calcitriol)
Cholecalciferol (vitamin D_3 from ultraviolet irradiated skin) and
ergocalciferol (vitamin D_2 from plants) are hydroxylated in the liver
to form 25 hydroxyvitamin D (calcidiol), which is inactive. This is
converted in the kidney to either 1 : 25 dihydroxyvitamin D (which
is active), or 24 : 25 dihydroxyvitamin D (which is inactive)

Actions of calcitriol
   (i)   Increases absorption of calcium and phosphate from the gut
  (ii)   Acts on bone to promote bone resorption

3. Calcitonin
Calcitonin is decreased in the short-term by a fall in blood calcium
Calcitonin is maintained in the long-term by oestrogen and testosterone

Action of calcitonin
Calcitonin decreases bone resorption by reducing the number and the activity of the osteoclasts. It thus opposes the resorptive actions of PTH and calcitriol

CALCITONIN (CT)

Synthesized mainly in C-cells of thyroid. CT opposes bone resorption, and also affects renal electrolyte excretion and milk composition
    Another peptide whose synthesis is governed by the same gene is calcitonin-gene-related peptide (CGRP), a potent vasodilator and a probable neurotransmitter

Causes of increased CT
  1. *Physiological*
     Infancy, pregnancy and lactation
  2. *Medullary carcinoma of thyroid*
  3. *Other tumours*, e.g. oat-cell Ca., breast Ca.,
     phaeochromocytoma, carcinoid
  4. *Myeloid leukaemia*
  5. *Miscellaneous*
     Vit. D metabolites
     Oral contraceptives
     Hyperparathyroidism
     Chronic lung disease
     Megaloblastic anaemia

Causes of decreased CT
  1. *Physiological*
     Lower in women than men, and decreases with age
  2. *Total thyroidectomy*
  3. *Gonadal failure*
  4. *Osteoporosis*
     (Postmenopause, but also some idiopathic cases)

METABOLIC BONE DISEASE

Osteomalacia is characterized by impaired bone mineralization with increased osteoid

Causes of osteomalacia and rickets
1. *Deficiency of cholecalciferol (vit. D)*
     (i)   Prematurity, multiple pregnancy, prolonged breast feeding and lack of UV predispose to rickets
    (ii)   Dietary
   (iii)   Post-gastrectomy (probably dietary)
    (iv)   Malabsorption
     (v)   Anticonvulsants (liver enzyme induction)
2. *Renal causes*
     (i)   Chronic renal failure
    (ii)   Idiopathic hypercalciuria
   (iii)   Fanconi syndrome
    (iv)   Tubular acidosis
3. *Hepatic disease (disturbed vit. D metabolism)*
4. *Hypophosphatasia*

Osteoporosis is characterized by reduced bone mass with normal mineralization

Causes of osteoporosis
1. Senile osteoporosis
2. Immobilization
3. Endocrine
      Sex hormone deficiency, e.g. premature menopause
      Cushing's or glucocorticoid therapy
      Hyperthyroidism
      Hyperparathyroidism
      Diabetes mellitus
4. Deficiency of oestrogen, androgen, protein, vit. C or calcium
5. Chronic renal failure
6. Miscellaneous
      Alcoholism
      Smoking
      Anticonvulsants
      Osteogenesis imperfecta
      Werner Rothmund syndrome
      Glycogen storage disease
      Cirrhosis in children
      Systemic mastocytosis or heparin infusion
      Homocystinuria
7. Localized osteoporosis, e.g. rheumatoid arthritis
8. Idiopathic osteoporosis of young people

Types of hepatic osteodystrophy
1. Osteomalacia (mainly due to lack of vitamin D substrate)
2. Osteoporosis
3. Periosteal reaction with new bone formation
4. Secondary hyperparathyroidism (very rare)

Renal osteodystrophy
Any cause of chronic renal failure can cause *increased phosphate excretion* and *decreased calcitriol synthesis*. These factors lead to parathyroid over-activity (osteitis fibrosa cystica) and defective bone mineralization. Aluminium toxicity (haemodialysis) may aggravate the osteomalacia

Causes of hypocalcaemia
1. Hypoparathyroidism
   (i) Post-thyroidectomy
   (ii) Idiopathic (sometimes with hypoadrenalism and Candidosis)
2. Deficiency of cholecalciferol
3. Malabsorption
4. Chronic renal failure or Fanconi syndrome (p. 173)
5. Hypoalbuminaemia
6. Neonatal hypocalcaemia
   (i) High-phosphate artificial feeds
   (ii) Associated with low birth-weight and hypoglycaemia
   (iii) Parathyroid suppression due to maternal hyperparathyroidism
7. 'Shock', e.g. septicaemia or acute pancreatitis
8. Malignancy, especially prostatic with osteosclerotic deposits
9. Cytotoxic drugs
10. Pseudo-hypoparathyroidism

Causes of hypercalcaemia
1. Hyperparathyroidism
2. Malignancy with or without metastases
3. Myelomatosis (rarely lymphoma or leukaemia)
4. Vit. D sensitivity, especially sarcoidosis
5. Vit. D excess
6. Milk-alkali syndrome
7. Drugs, e.g. thiazides, lithium
8. Thyrotoxicosis
9. Hypothyroidism, especially in infants
10. Infantile hypercalcaemia
11. Acute renal failure in polyuric phase
12. Steroid withdrawal (iatrogenic, or acute hypoadrenalism)
13. Paget's disease (when immobilized)
14. Immobilization (very rarely)

Causes of hypercalciuria
1. All causes of hypercalcaemia, if renal function is normal
2. Renal tubular acidosis
3. Progressive osteoporosis
4. Cushing's syndrome
5. Acromegaly
6. Prolonged immobilization
7. Excess dietary calcium
8. Idiopathic hypercalciuria

Causes of hypophosphataemia
Primary
Hyperparathyroidism
Osteomalacia
Renal tubular acidosis
Iatrogenic   Excess phosphate binders, renal failure patients
TPN without correct supplementation
Treatment of diabetic ketoacidosis
Feeding in anorexics after starvation
Post dialysis
Recovery from burns
Malnutrition

Causes of hyperphosphataemia
Renal failure
Hypoparathyroidism
Pseudohypoparathyroidism

Tests to distinguish hyperparathyroidism from other causes of hypercalcaemia
1. *Steroid suppression test*
   Hypercalcaemia due to hyperparathyroidism is not suppressed by cortisol 40 mg tds
2. *Plasma phosphate*
   Consistently low PO_4 suggests primary hyperparathyroidism
3. *Phosphate excretion tests* (e.g. PEI, p. 239)
   Based on blockage of net phosphate reabsorption by parathormone
4. *Acid-base status*
   Patients with hyperparathyroidism have hyperchloraemic acidosis
   Other hypercalcaemic patients have hypochloraemic alkalosis
5. *Parathormone radioimmunoassay*
6. *Plasma alkaline phosphatase*
   Increased in patients with X-ray signs of hyperparathyroidism (osteoblastic activity)

7. *Calcium tolerance tests* (urinary phosphate excretion after calcium infusion)
Parathormone production is not suppressed in hyperparathyroidism. Of limited value due to false positives and negatives

Causes of soft-tissue calcification
1. *Dystrophic*
Occurs in abnormal tissue, often with impaired blood supply
   (i)   Inflammatory foci, e.g. TB
   (ii) Neoplasia and naevi
   (iii) Parasites, e.g. cysticercosis
   (iv) Haematoma
   (v)   Gravitational oedema (esp. leg ulcers)
   (vi) Systemic sclerosis, dermatomyositis
   (vii) Ehlers–Danlos syndrome (cutis hyperelastica)
2. *Metastatic (metabolic)*
Calcification of normal tissue, e.g. kidneys or arteries, due to a metabolic abnormality such as hypercalcaemia or hypervitaminosis D. Intracranial calcification occurs in hypoparathyroidism and pseudohypoparathyroidism
3. *Secondary to bone or joint disease*
e.g. calcified cartilage, tendon or periosteum
4. *Idiopathic calcification*
   (i)   Calcinosis circumscripta
   (ii) Calcinosis universalis
   (iii) Myositis ossificans

Causes of discrete translucences in a skull X-ray
1. Hyperparathyroidism
2. Myelomatosis
3. Metastatic deposits, esp. neuroblastoma
4. Leukaemia
5. Sickle-cell anaemia
6. Langerhans cell histiocytosis, esp. Hand–Schuller-Christian disease
7. Sarcoidosis
8. Congenital cranial lacunae

Causes of bilateral frontal 'bossing'
1. Paget's
2. Rickets
3. Achondroplasia
4. Congenital hydrocephalus
5. Basal cell naevi syndrome (Gorlin's)

Causes of 'bowing' of tibia
1. Paget's
2. Rickets
3. Syphilis or yaws
4. Polyostotic fibrous dysplasia (Albright's)

Renal disease

CAUSES OF CHRONIC RENAL FAILURE

In order of percentage frequency in Europe
Glomerulonephritis 33%
Pyelonephritis 21%
Unknown cause 10%
Cystic kidney disease 9%
Multisystem (e.g. diabetes mellitus, amyloid) 9%
Renal vascular disease 8%
Drug nephropathy 3%
Other causes 7%
In some other areas malarial nephropathy, schistosomiasis and sickle-cell disease are important

DIALYSIS

Possible indications for short-term dialysis
1. Acute renal failure
    (i)   Hyperkalaemia > 7 mmol/l
    (ii) Arterial pH < 7.15
    (iii) Blood urea > 35 mmol/l
    (iv) Rapidly rising blood urea
2. Fluid overload
3. Uncontrolled hypercalcaemia
4. Gross electrolyte disturbance
5. Poisoning with salicylates
                  barbiturates
                  ethanol
6. Acute-on-chronic renal failure prior to establishing conservative therapy

Possible indications for long-term haemodialysis
1. Failure of conservative management
2. Serum creatinine > 1200 μmol/l
3. GFR < 3 ml/min
4. Progression of bone disease

5. Progression of neuropathy
6. Onset of pericarditis (peritoneal dialysis may be necessary initially to avoid haemopericarditis)

Complications of haemodialysis

A.   *Acute and subacute*
1. Infection, via shunt or extracorporeal circulation
2. Cardiovascular
    (i)   Hypotension or hypertension
    (ii) Angina
    (iii) Dysrhythmia
    (iv) Heart failure and fluid overload
3. Haematological
    (i)   Leukopenia (severe, transient)
    (ii) Thrombocytopenia (mild, progressive)
    (iii) Complement activation
    (iv) Haemorrhage
    (v)   Haemolysis (rare)
4. Respiratory
        Hypoxaemia (usually mild)
5. Electrolyte
    (i)   Hypokalaemia (during dialysis)
    (ii) Hyperkalaemia (between dialyses)
    (iii) Hyponatraemia or hypernatraemia
    (iv) Hard water syndrome (hypercalcaemia, hypermagnesaemia)
6. Neurological
    (i)   Stroke (haemorrhage, embolism, hypotension)
    (ii) Disequilibrium syndrome (raised c.s.f. pressure)
    (iii) Hypertensive encephalopathy
7. Miscellaneous
    (i)   Febrile reactions
    (ii) Air embolism
    (iii) Anaphylaxis
    (iv) Intravenous formaldehyde (pain and coughing)
    (v)   Priapism

B.   *Chronic*
1. Anaemia
    Loss of erythropoietin, reduced RBC survival, loss during dialysis, dietary deficiency, venesection, aluminium toxicity, etc.
2. Cardiovascular
    (i)   Hypertension
    (ii) Cardiac ischaemia
    (iii) Peripheral vascular disease
    (iv) Fistula thrombosis

3. Neurological
   (i)   Dialysis dementia (aluminium intoxication)
   (ii) Peripheral neuropathy
   (iii) Carpal tunnel syndrome
   (iv) Thiamine deficiency
4. Osteodystrophic
   (i)   Hyperparathyroidism
   (ii) Osteomalacia
   (iii) Aluminium-induced bone disease (osteomalacia with multiple fractures)
5. Metabolic
   Disorders of hormones (increased MSH, glucagon, GH, gastrin) and lipids (esp. raised triglycerides with type IV hyperlipidaemia)
6. Sexual
   Disorders affecting fertility, potency and pregnancy
7. Psychological (increased suicide risk)
8. Hepatitis (esp. B, and C)
9. Cancer risk increased
10. Trace element accumulation, (e.g. silicon from blood pump tubing can cause hepatic fibromas)

Continuous peritoneal ambulatory dialysis (CAPD)

Advantages of CAPD over regular haemodialysis
1. Simple technique (no machinery, alarms, etc.)
2. Causes less fluctuation in blood pressure, fluid balance and biochemistry
3. Diet less restrictive
4. Patient more mobile and independent
5. Many patients are less anaemic

Complications of CAPD
1. Poor flow of dialysate
2. Leakage of dialysate fluid along insertion track
3. Infection
   (i)   Local, around the cuff
   (ii) Peritonitis, may be bacterial or fungal
   (iii) Subacute sclerosing peritonitis
4. Hernia formation, may be incisional, inguinal, periumbilical or hiatus hernia

Renal causes of polycythaemia
1. Hypernephroma
2. Polycystic disease
3. Hydronephrosis
4. Renal artery stenosis
5. Transplantation

GLOMERULONEPHRITIS

Histological classification
1. *Minimal lesion* (no change on light microscopy)
2. *Membranous* (no cellular proliferation)
3. *Proliferative glomerulonephritis (PGN)*
   Each of the 3 cellular elements, epithelial, endothelial or mesangial, may show proliferative changes together or singly
   (i) Active diffuse endothelial PGN
   (ii) Mesangial PGN
   (iii) Rapidly progressive PGN with extensive epithelial crescents
   (iv) Mesangiocapillary PGN
   (v) Focal PGN (affects only some parts of some glomeruli)
   (vi) Chronic endothelial PGN
4. *Focal glomerulosclerosis*
5. *Advanced sclerosing lesions*
   3(i) and 3(ii) are commonly post-streptococcal

Clinical syndromes of glomerulonephritis
1. Acute nephritis
2. Nephrotic syndrome
3. Persistent proteinuria
4. Recurrent haematuria or loin pain
5. Chronic renal failure
6. Acute oliguric renal failure (rare)

Antigens implicated in glomerulonephritis
1. *Bacterial*
   Streptococcal (β haemolytic, type 12)
   Staphylococci (in bact. endocarditis and in 'shunt' nephritis)
   Mycobact. leprae
   Treponema pallidum
   Salmonella typhi
   Yersinia
2. *Viral*
   Hepatitis B and C, HIV, varicella, measles, mumps, EB virus, Coxsackie B
3. *Protozoal*
   Plasmodium malariae, schistosoma, toxoplasma
4. *Worms*
   Loaiasis, filariasis
5. *Others*
   DNA (in SLE)
   Thyroglobulin (in autoimmune thyroiditis)
   Cryoglobulin
   Tumour antigens
   Carcinoembryonic antigen (in Ca. colon)
   Drugs, e.g. penicillamine, heroin, mercury, gold

CAUSES OF NEPHROTIC SYNDROME
1. *Glomerulonephritis* (p. 168)
   Accounts for 80% of cases
2. *Metabolic*
   (i)   Diabetes mellitus
   (ii) Amyloidosis
   (iii) Lymphoma
   (iv) Extrarenal malignancy, e.g. bronchus
   (v)   Dysproteinaemia, esp. myelomatosis
   (vi) Dermatoses
   (vii) Sickle-cell anaemia
   (viii) Myxoedema
3. *'Collagen-vascular' disease*
   esp. SLE and vasculitis
4. *Infection*
   (i)   Malaria
   (ii) Cytomegalic inclusion disease
   (iii) Syphilis
   (iv) Bacterial endocarditis
   (v)   Staphylococcal septicaemia
   (vi) Leprosy
5. *Mechanical*
   Renal artery stenosis
   Renal vein thrombosis (may be cause or effect)
   Inf. vena caval thrombosis
   Constrictive pericarditis
   Renal carcinoma
   Chyluria
6. *Drugs*
   Mercurials, troxidone, penicillamine, gold, etc.
7. *Hypersensitivity*
   (i) Serum sickness, bee stings, poison ivy, pollen, etc.
   (ii) Smallpox vaccination
8. *Congenital and familial*

Causes of renal vein thrombosis
1. Nephrotic syndrome of any cause
2. Renal amyloid
3. Hypernephroma
4. Trauma, including cannulation
5. Dehydration, especially in infancy

Causes of papillary necrosis
1. Analgesic abuse, esp. phenacetin
2. Obstructive uropathy, esp. with infection
3. Acute pyelonephritis, esp. in diabetes mellitus
4. Sickle-cell disease

5. Renal TB
6. Dysproteinaemia

Chronic interstitial nephritis
Defined as renal disease with the histological features of chronic
pyelonephritis but with no evidence of bacterial infection. The
condition is underdiagnosed, but is becoming more important with
the increasing use of nephrotoxic drugs. Sterile pyuria in the
absence of urinary tract TB should suggest the possibility

Causes of interstitial nephritis
1. Drugs
        Analgesics (esp. phenacetin abuse)
        Anticonvulsants
        Anticoagulants
        Antibacterials
        NSAIDs
        Cytotoxics
2. Chemicals and toxins
        Cadmium, lead or lithium
        Balkan nephropathy (due to fungal toxin)
3. Metabolic
        Hypokalaemia
        Hyperuricaemia
        Nephrocalcinosis
4. Immunological damage
        Kidney graft rejection
        Sjøgren's syndrome
        Methicillin nephritis
5. Physical or mechanical
        X-irradiation
        Reflux nephropathy
6. Vascular damage
        Diabetes mellitus
        'Ageing kidney'
        Sickle-cell disease
7. Congenital
        Alport's disease
        Medullary cystic disease
        Nephronophthisis

Causes of 'sterile' pyuria
1. Renal TB
2. Analgesic nephropathy
3. Renal calculi
4. Urinary infection treated with chemotherapy
5. Drugs
        (i) Analgesics

  (ii) Diuretics
  (iii) Iron sorbitol citric acid complex (Jectofer)
6. Non-specific urethritis

NEPHROCALCINOSIS AND RENAL STONES

Causes of renal stones
1. *Calcium stones* (oxalate, phosphate, mixed magnesium-ammonium, etc.)
   (i) With hypercalcaemia
       Primary hyperparathyroidism
       Sarcoidosis
       Idiopathic hypercalcaemia of infancy
       Chronic milk-alkali syndrome
       Vit. D excess
   (ii) With normocalcaemia
       Idiopathic hypercalciuria
       Prolonged bed rest
       Primary renal tubular acidosis
       Urinary tract infection
       Hyperoxaluria
       Medullary sponge kidney
2. *Uric acid stones*
   (i) With hyperuricaemia
       Gout
       Polycythaemia, leukaemia, malignancy, etc.
       Chronic metabolic acidosis, e.g. glycogen storage disease
       Lesch–Nyhan syndrome
   (ii) With normouricaemia
       Idiopathic
       Acid, concentrated urine (e.g. desert climates)
3. *Cystine stones*
   (i) Congenital cystinuria
   (ii) Hereditary cystinosis
4. *Xanthine stones* Xanthinuria

Radio-opaque stones	Non-opaque stones
Calcium	Uric acid
Mg-ammonium phosphate	Xanthine
Cystine	Matrix
Silicate	

Differential diagnosis
Blood clot
Sloughed papillae
Tumour
Varices

Radiographic nephrocalcinosis

1. *Coarse, medullary*

Causes
- (i) Primary hyperparathyroidism
- (ii) Primary renal tubular acidosis
- (iii) Sarcoidosis
- (iv) Milk-alkali syndrome
- (v) Primary hyperoxaluria (oxalosis)
- (vi) Idiopathic hypercalcuria
- (vii) Idiopathic

2. *Localized*

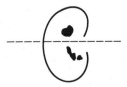

Causes
- (i) Medullary sponge kidney (calcified collecting ducts)
- (ii) Renal neoplasm
- (iii) Cyst or haematoma
- (iv) Papillary necrosis
- (v) TB
- (vi) Hydatid cyst

3. *Diffuse, cortical (Rare)*

Causes
- (i) Chronic glomerulonephritis
- (ii) Old cortical necrosis

Causes of small kidneys
1. Chronic glomerulonephritis (smooth outline)
2. Chronic pyelonephritis (irregular outline)
3. Other chronic nephropathy, e.g. interstitial nephritis
4. Renal artery stenosis
5. Atrophy following obstruction
6. Congenital renal hypoplasia (prone to infection)

Causes of large kidney (or kidneys)
1. Cystic kidneys (q.v.)
2. Hydronephrosis or pyonephrosis
3. Hypernephroma
4. Hypertrophy following contralateral nephrectomy or failure
5. Nephrotic syndrome
6. Acute pyelonephritis
7. Compulsive water, beer or cider drinker

Also consider the possibility of perirenal haematoma

Cystic kidneys

Causes
1. *Polycystic kidney*
   (i)   Adult form (autosomal dominant)
   (ii) Infantile form (autosomal recessive)
2. *Multicystic kidney*
   Usually functionless and associated with atresia or absence of ureter
3. *Nephronophthisis-cystic renal medulla complex*
   Characterized clinically by polyuria and urinary salt-wasting
   Three types:
   (i)   Familial juvenile (autosomal recessive)
   (ii) Retinal (esp. with retinitis pigmentosa)
   (iii) Medullary cysts (autosomal dominant)
4. *Medullary sponge kidney*
   Often complicated by calculi or pyelonephritis
5. *Simple renal cysts*
   Often multiple, and usually asymptomatic
6. *Miscellaneous*
   Renal cysts can also occur in a wide variety of other diseases, e.g. endometriosis, echinococcal disease, TB, neoplasm, etc.

RENAL TUBULAR DISORDERS

Single transport defects
1. *Impaired reabsorption*
   Water—nephrogenic diabetes insipidus
   Na or K—distal tubular damage, e.g. chronic pyelonephritis
   Calcium—idiopathic hypercalciuria
   Phosphate—vitamin D resistant rickets
   Glucose—renal glycosuria
   Amino acids—see page 174
   Xanthine—xanthinuria
2. *Excessive reabsorption*
   Phosphate—pseudohypoparathyroidism

Multiple transport defects
1. *Impaired acidification*
   (i)   Renal tubular acidosis
   (ii) Chronic pyelonephritis
   (iii) Hypokalaemia
   (iv) Hypercalcaemia
   (v)   Hydronephrosis
2. *Impaired reabsorption and acidification*
   (Fanconi syndrome) e.g.
   (i)   Hereditary cystinosis (Lignac–Fanconi)
   (ii) Toxins—cadmium, Hg, lead

　(iii)　Drugs—neomycin, outdated tetracycline
　(iv)　Galactosaemia
　　(v)　Hepatolenticular degeneration
　(vi)　Nephrotic syndrome
　(vii)　Lowe's oculo-cerebro-renal syndrome

AMINO-ACIDURIA

Four groups with separate transport systems
1. Proline, hydroxyproline and glycine
2. Dibasic: cystine, ornithine, arginine and lysine (COAL)
3. Dicarboxylic: glutamic and aspartic acids
4. Monoamino-monocarboxylic: all the rest

Causes of amino-aciduria
1. *Pure 'overflow'* due to raised plasma levels
   Amino-acid infusion
   Liver failure
   Phenylketonuria
   Maple-syrup urine
   Histidinaemia
   Glycinaemia
2. *A specific transport defect*
   Cystinuria
   Hartnup disease (malabsorption, ataxia and pellagrous rash)
3. *Generalized proximal tubular damage* (Fanconi syndrome)
4. *Mixed 'overflow' and renal*
   Citrullinuria
   Prolinaemia

SOME CAUSES OF 'DARK COLOURED' URINE
1. Concentration
2. Bile
3. Blood, haemoglobinuria or myoglobinuria
4. Methaemoglobinuria
5. Porphyria
6. Alkaptonuria
7. Melaninuria
8. Beetroot, dyes in sweets, drugs, e.g. PAS

Important causes of haemoglobinuria
1. *Autoimmune haemolysis*
   Paroxysmal cold haemoglobinuria
   Cold haemagglutinin disease
2. *Nonimmune haemolysis*
   March haemoglobinuria
   Paroxysmal nocturnal haemoglobinuria

Sickle-cell crisis
Falciparum malaria (Blackwater fever)
Extensive burns

DRUG-INDUCED RENAL DISEASE

1. **Acute renal failure**
   (20% of cases are due to drugs)
   Over 70 drugs implicated, and a variety of mechanisms
     (i)   Direct toxicity (dose-related)
           e.g. cephaloridine, amphotericin B, cyclosporin A
     (ii) Hypersensitivity
           e.g. penicillin, sulphonamides
     (iii) Obstruction due to crystal formation
           e.g. sulphonamides
     (iv) 'Osmotic nephrosis'
           e.g. low MW dextran infusion
   Acute tubular necrosis may be due to aminoglycosides, cyclosporin or radiographic contrast media
   Interstitial nephritis may be due to NSAIDs or penicillin
   Tetracyclines cause two distinct disorders:
     a. Renal failure (due to increased urea production, increased sodium excretion and reduced urine-concentrating ability)
     b. Degraded tetracyclines cause proximal tubular defects (Fanconi syndrome)

2. **Drug-induced LE**
   (especially in slow acetylators)

3. **Nephrotic syndrome**

4. **Papillary necrosis**
   Analgesics, especially phenacetin

5. **Retroperitoneal fibrosis**
   e.g. methysergide, ergotamine, methyldopa

6. **Metabolic effects**
     (i)   Increased protein breakdown, e.g. glucocorticoids
     (ii) Electrolyte disturbance, e.g. drugs causing diarrhoea
     (iii) Nephrocalcinosis, e.g. vitamin D overdosage
     (iv) Renal calculi, e.g. 'milk-alkali' syndrome
     (v)   Urate nephropathy, e.g. cytotoxins for malignancy
     (vi) Impaired urine-concentrating ability, e.g.
           demethylchlortetracycline, lithium
     (vii) Inappropriate ADH secretion

7. **Neoplasm**
   Renal pelvis mesothelial tumour, e.g. analgesics

8. **Vascular**
   ACE inhibitors may provoke renal artery thrombosis in pre-existing mild renal artery stenosis

RENAL DISEASE DUE TO ENVIRONMENTAL TOXINS

Causes
1. *Metals*
   Arsenic, cadmium, lead, mercury, silicon
2. *Hydrocarbons*
   Petroleum products and organic solvents
3. *Herbicides,* especially Paraquat
4. *Plant and animal toxins*
   Fungi (especially *Amanita phalloides*), snake venom, multiple bee stings

ACID-BASE BALANCE

These headings reflect changes in extracellular fluid only, e.g. in metabolic alkalosis there is an associated intracellular acidosis
1. RESPIRATORY ACIDOSIS (Low pH, High CO_2 content)
   Any cause of hypoventilation (p. 25)
2. RESPIRATORY ALKALOSIS (High pH, Low CO_2 content)
   Any cause of hyperventilation (p. 26)
3. METABOLIC ACIDOSIS (Low pH, Low CO_2 content)
   Causes
   (i) *Ingestion of hydrion or 'potential acid'*
       Diets high in protein and fat
       Ammonium chloride, salicylates, calcium chloride, etc.
       'Dilution acidaemia' due to rapid saline infusion
   (ii) *Metabolic overproduction of hydrions*
        Hypercatabolic states
        Ketosis, e.g. starvation, diabetes mellitus
        Lactic acidosis (p. 177)
   (iii) *Intestinal loss of base*
         Diarrhoea
         Fistulae
   (iv) *Renal causes*
        a. Acute or chronic failure
        b. Defective hydrion secretion
            Renal tubular acidosis
            Pyelonephritis
            Hydronephrosis
        c. Extrarenal causes
            Carbonic anhydrase inhibitors
            Addison's disease
            Ureterosigmoidostomy

4. METABOLIC ALKALOSIS (High pH, High CO_2 content)
   Causes
   Ingestion of alkali, e.g. $NaHCO_3$
   Vomiting, or gastric aspiration
   Hypokalaemia (see below)
5. MIXED DISORDERS
   e.g. Respiratory and metabolic acidosis in hypoventilated
       hypoxic patients
       Respiratory alkalosis and metabolic acidosis in salicylate
       poisoning

LACTIC ACIDOSIS

Metabolic acidosis with blood pH < 7.25 and serum lactate >
5 mmol/l

Causes of lactic acidosis
1. *Poor tissue perfusion or hypoxia,* e.g. 'shock'
2. *Metabolic disease*
       Renal failure
       Hepatic failure
       Infection
       Diabetic ketoacidosis
       Pancreatitis
       Leukaemia or lymphoma
3. *Drugs*
       Phenformin or metformin
       Ethanol or methanol
       Fructose, etc.
4. *Ingestion of 'lactic acid' milk*
5. *Congenital*
       G6P deficiency, etc.
NB An increased anion gap $([Na^+] + [K^+]) - ([Cl^-] + [HCO_3^-])$ is
helpful in diagnosis if blood lactate estimation cannot be performed
(normal anion gap 10–18 mmol/l)

Causes of hypokalaemia
1. *Increased renal loss*
   (i) Diuresis
       Drugs
       Diabetes mellitus
   (ii) Minerolocorticoid excess
       Primary aldosteronism (Conn's tumour)
       Cushing's
       Ingestion of liquorice or carbenoxolone
   (iii) Primary renal disease
       Diuretic phase of acute renal failure
       Chronic pyelonephritis

Fanconi syndrome (p. 173)
Renal tubular acidosis
Renal ischaemia
2. *Increased intestinal loss*
Diarrhoea
Vomiting
Aspiration
Fistulae
Resonium A
3. *Decreased intake*
Dietary lack (especially in alcoholism, or during protein anabolism in convalescence)
Malabsorption
4. *Familial periodic paralysis*
5. *IV insulin*
6. *Severe asthma,* due to β-agonists, glucocorticoids and hypoxia

Causes of hypokalaemic acidosis
NB *Alkalosis is more usual*
1. Pancreatic fistulae (loss of HCO_3)
2. Vipoma
3. Renal tubular acidosis
4. Ureteric implants into the sigmoid colon

Causes of hypernatraemia
1. *Inadequate water intake*
Lack of water, inability to drink, etc.
2. *Inadequate water retention*
Diabetes insipidus
3. *Excessive sodium intake*
Diet or drugs (oral or intravenous)
4. *Excessive sodium retention*
Hyperaldosteronism

Causes of hyponatraemia
1. *Excessive water intake*
Oral (polydipsia) or intravenous
2. *Excessive water retention*
Inappropriate ADH secretion
3. *Inadequate sodium intake* (rare)
4. *Inadequate sodium retention*
   (i)   Vomiting, diarrhoea, ileus, fistula, drainage of ascites
   (ii) Hypoadrenalism
   (iii) Renal
         a. Salt-losing nephropathy
         b. Osmotic diuresis
         c. Excessive diuretic therapy

(iv) Skin
   a. Excessive sweating
   b. Cystic fibrosis
   c. Burns

Drugs causing sodium and water retention
1. Corticosteroids and corticotrophin, e.g. fludrocortisone
2. Oestrogens
3. Anti-inflammatory drugs, e.g. phenylbutazone
4. Carbenoxolone and liquorice-like compounds
5. Vasodilators, e.g. minoxidil, diazoxide
6. Hypotensives (esp. at start of therapy), e.g. guanethidine
7. Psychotropic drugs, e.g. lithium
8. Sodium-containing drugs, e.g. liquid antacids
                                        carbenecillin
                                        X-ray contrast media

Causes of hypomagnesaemia
1. Inadequate dietary intake (rare)
2. Malabsorption or loss from GI tract (diarrhoea, fistula, etc.)
3. Excessive urinary loss
   (i) Drugs—diuretics, aminoglycosides, cisplatin
   (ii) Alcoholism
   (iii) With nephrocalcinosis
4. Endocrine
   (i) Diabetic ketoacidosis
   (ii) Hyperparathyroidism

CAUSES OF POLYDIPSIA AND POLYURIA
1. *Decreased vasopressin production*
   (i) Cranial diabetes insipidus
        Congenital
        Head injury or neurosurgery
        Tumours, e.g. craniopharyngioma
        Sarcoid, Langerhans, histiocytosis X, TB, etc.
   (ii) Psychogenic polydipsia
2. *Decreased renal tubular response to vasopressin*
   (i) Congenital nephrogenic diabetes insipidus
   (ii) Hypercalcaemia or hypokalaemia
   (iii) Chronic renal failure
   (iv) Obstructive uropathy
   (v) Lithium therapy, demeclocycline
   (vi) Psychogenic polydipsia
3. *Osmotic diuresis*
   (i) Heavy glycosuria
   (ii) Mannitol therapy

4. *Dry mouth*
   Sjögren's syndrome

ARGININE VASOPRESSIN (Antidiuretic hormone)

Causes of inappropriate ADH secretion
1. *Neoplasm*
   Ectopic synthesis, especially bronchial oat-cell Ca., but also leukaemia, lymphoma, sarcoma, etc.
2. *Neurohypophyseal disease*
   Intracranial inflammation, bleeding, tumour, trauma, etc.
3. *Non-neoplastic thoracic disease*
   TB, pneumonia, cardiac surgery, asthma, IPPV, pneumothorax
4. *Endocrine*
   Hypoadrenalism, hypothyroidism, hypopituitarism, hypoglycaemia, stress
5. *Metabolic*
   Alcoholism
   Porphyria
6. *Drugs*
   Barbiturates   Thiazides
   Carbamazepine   Amitryptiline
   Cyclophosphamide   Chlorpropamide
   Clofibrate   Indomethacin
   Nicotine   Vincristine
7. *Miscellaneous*
   Pain, trauma, hypotension

Criteria for diagnosis of inappropriate ADH secretion
1. Hyponatraemia with reduced plasma osmolality
2. Continued sodium excretion
3. Normal extracellular fluid volume
4. Urine not maximally dilute
5. Normal renal and adrenal function

Rheumatology

Radiological features

Osteoarthrosis
1. New bone formation
    Osteophytes
    Periarticular ossicles
    Loose bodies
2. Joint space narrowing due to cartilage loss
3. Sclerosis and subchondral cavitation
4. Juxta-articular cysts
5. Subluxation in advanced cases
6. **No** ankylosis

Ankylosing spondylitis
1. Bilateral erosive SI disease, with later sclerosis
2. Erosion in intervertebral facets and costovertebral joints
3. Calcified spinal ligaments
4. Erosion in limb joints, especially hips
5. Irregularity of weight-bearing surfaces
6. Calcification of the entheses

Rheumatoid arthritis
1. Juxta-articular osteoporosis
2. Cartilage loss
3. Marginal and surface erosions
4. Subluxations, dislocations and carpal ankylosis
5. **No** sclerosis or new bone formation

Chondrocalcinosis
Calcium deposits (punctate-linear opacities) are seen esp. in AP view of knees, and in symphysis pubis and wrists

Gout
In acute gout, no change
In chronic gout, juxta-articular bony destruction causes typical punched-out lesions, with surrounding calcification

Paget's disease
Variable, but diagnostic:
1. Areas of resorption or osteolysis
2. Areas of thickening or sclerosis
3. Deformity

Osteoporosis
1. Loss of bone density when compared with standard films of normal bones
2. Wedge collapse of vertebral bodies
3. Apparent increase in density of vertebral end-plates

Osteomalacia
1. Increased lucency of bones (osteopenia)
2. 'Looser zones' (pseudofractures) due to uncalcified osteoid seams, especially in femoral neck, pubic bones, ribs and scapulae
3. Collapse of lumbar vertebrae
4. Bowing or distortion of weight-bearing bones

Causes of bone pain
1. Malignancy (esp. myeloma) or metastasis
2. Congenital haemolytic anaemia (especially sickle-cell disease)
3. Myelofibrosis
4. Hodgkin's disease (esp. after alcohol)

Causes of a periosteal reaction
1. Osteomyelitis
2. Healing fracture
3. Juvenile chronic arthritis
4. Hypertrophic pulmonary osteoarthropathy
5. Psoriatic arthritis
6. Reiter's syndrome
7. Cellulitis
8. Bone tumours, e.g. osteosarcoma
9. Subperiosteal haemorrhage, e.g. scurvy
10. Polyarteritis nodosa
11. Thyroid acropachy
12. Pachydermoperiostitis

Causes of lumbar backache
1. *Mechanical*
   (i)   Musculotendinous and ligament strain
   (ii) Prolapsed intervertebral disc
   (iii) Spondylosis and spondylolisthesis

    (iv) Spinal fracture
- a. Major trauma
- b. Crush fracture in osteoporosis
- c. Stress fracture of transverse process due to muscular effort

    (v) Segmental instability
    (vi) Congenital anomaly, e.g. sacralization of L5, scoliosis

2. *Degenerative or metabolic*
   - (i) Osteoarthrosis
   - (ii) Paget's disease
   - (iii) Osteoporosis with fracture
   - (iv) Osteomalacia and renal osteodystrophy
   - (v) Diffuse idiopathic skeletal hyperostosis (DISH)
   - (vi) Ochronosis (alkaptonuria)

3. *Inflammatory*
   - (i) Infection
     - a. Pyogenic infection (esp. *Staph. aureus* or Gm. negative bacilli)
     - b. TB
     - c. Brucellosis
     - d. Salmonella, with osteomyelitis or paravertebral abscess
   - (ii) Seronegative spondyloarthritis (q.v.)
   - (iii) Scheuermann's disease (osteochondritis of vertebral end-plates)

4. *Neoplasm*
   - (i) Usually metastatic malignancy
   - (ii) Primary malignancy—Osteosarcoma
                              Myeloma
                              Lymphoma
   - (iii) Rarely, benign tumour (e.g. neurofibroma)

5. *Referred pain*
   - (i) Posterior duodenal ulcer
   - (ii) Cancer of pancreas
   - (iii) Renal colic
   - (iv) Pelvic carcinoma
   - (v) Dysmenorrhoea, labour pains
   - (vi) Retroperitoneal haematoma

SERONEGATIVE SPONDYLOARTHRITIS

Arthritis involving the spine but with consistent absence of rheumatoid factors from serum
1. Ankylosing spondylitis
2. Psoriatic arthritis
3. Enteropathic arthritis (Crohn's, ulcerative colitis, Whipple's, enteric infection, intestinal bypass for obesity)

4. Reiter's disease
5. Behçet's disease

Patterns of psoriatic arthritis
1. Predominant distal interphalangeal arthritis
2. Severe deforming arthritis with widespread ankylosis ('arthritis mutilans')
3. Mimicking benign rheumatoid arthritis, but consistently seronegative
4. Asymmetrical oligoarthritis (i.e. one or a few joints only)
5. Spondylitis or sacroiliitis

OSTEOARTHROSIS

Causes

A. *Primary (idiopathic)*

B. *Secondary*
  1. Mechanical
    (i) Previous orthopaedic problems. May be congenital (e.g. hip dislocation) or acquired (e.g. malaligned fracture, post-meniscectomy, slipped femoral epiphysis)
    (ii) Excessive 'wear and tear'
       Occupational, e.g. farmers and hip OA
       Obesity
       Long leg arthropathy
       Old rickets
  2. Hormonal and metabolic
     Acromegaly
     Haemochromatosis
     Ochronosis
     Familial chondrocalcinosis
     Kashin–Beck disease (seen in Eastern Europe due to ingestion of wheat contaminated with fungus)
  3. Pre-existing inflammatory disease
     Rheumatoid arthritis
     Gout
     Pseudo-gout

CALCIUM PYROPHOSPHATE ARTHROPATHY

Pseudo-gout (chondrocalcinosis) may mimic gout, rheumatoid arthritis, osteoarthrosis or neuropathic arthropathy
Numerous crystals (CPPD) in synovial fluid are diagnostic. X-rays may show chondrocalcinosis

Crystals of sodium urate are long and thin, while CPPD crystals are shorter and fatter. Under polarizing light, *urate* crystals show *negative* birefringence, whereas CPPD crystals are weakly positive

ASSOCIATED CONDITIONS

1. **Metabolic**
   Hyperuricaemia (with or without gout)
   Hyperparathyroidism
   Hepatolenticular degeneration (Wilson's)
   Haemochromatosis
   Ochronosis
   Hypophosphatasia
   Hypomagnesaemia
   Hypothyroidism

2. **Familial**

3. **Secondary**
   Surgery
   Trauma
   Hypermobility (p. 187)
   Other arthropathies, e.g. OA

4. **Idiopathic** (age-related)

CAUSES OF HYPERURICAEMIA

1. **Increased purine synthesis**
   (i)   Primary gout (in 25% of cases)
   (ii) Lesch–Nyhan syndrome (congenital mental deficiency, choreoathetosis and lip chewing)
   (iii) Mild HGPRT deficiency (i.e. partial form of Lesch–Nyhan)

2. **Increased turnover of preformed purines**
   (i)   Myeloproliferative disease and lymphoma
   (ii) Chronic haemolysis
   (iii) Psoriasis
   (iv) Fructose ingestion
   (v)   High purine diet

3. **Decreased renal excretion**
   (i)   Primary gout (in 75% of cases)
   (ii) Chronic renal failure
   (iii) Hyperparathyroidism
   (iv) Lead nephropathy
   (v)   Down's syndrome

(vi)   Increased organic acid production:
     Exercise
     Starvation, vomiting
     Diabetic ketoacidosis
     Alcohol
     Toxaemia of pregnancy
     Glycogen storage disease (G6P deficiency)
     Hyperlipidaemia
(vii)   Drugs
     Salicylates (in low dosage)
     Uricosurics (in low dosage)
     Diuretics
     Pyrazinamide
     Ethambutol

Serum uric acid also tends to be high in patients with hypertension, hyperlipidaemia, obesity and high IQ

CAUSES OF A TRANSIENT 'FLITTING' ARTHRITIS

1. Rheumatic fever
2. Henoch–Schönlein purpura
3. Serum sickness and drug reactions
4. SLE
5. Systemic infections
   (i)   Gonococcal or meningococcal septicaemia
  (ii)   Bacterial endocarditis
 (iii)   Rubella
 (iv)   Infectious mononucleosis
  (v)   Infective hepatitis
 (vi)   *Mycoplasma pneumonia*
6. Reiter's disease
7. Occasionally, acute rheumatoid arthritis or Still's disease

CAUSES OF A SINGLE HOT RED JOINT

1. Traumatic, e.g. sprained ankle
2. Septic arthritis
   May be secondary to penetrating injury, osteomyelitis, septicaemia, rheumatoid arthritis or osteoarthrosis
3. Gout or pseudo-gout (chondrocalcinosis or periarticular calcification)
4. Haemophilia
5. Gonococcal arthritis
6. Seronegative spondarthritis
7. Occasionally rheumatoid arthritis

INFECTIVE ARTHRITIS

Factors predisposing to joint infection
1. Previous arthritis (RA, OA, etc.)
2. General debility or severe systemic illness, e.g. alcoholism, malignancy, uraemia, diabetes mellitus, SLE
3. Immunosuppression
   e.g. AIDS, glucocorticoids, cytotoxic drugs, etc.
4. Sickle-cell disease (via osteomyelitis)
5. IV drug abuse
6. Infective focus elsewhere
   TB, bronchiectasis, skin sepsis, etc.
7. Orthopaedic procedures, e.g. arthroplasty

Organisms commonly found in infective arthritis
1. Staphylococci
2. Streptococci (including pneumococci)
3. *Haemophilus influenzae* (in children)
4. *E. coli*
5. *Neisseria gonorrhoeae*
6. *Neisseria meningitidis*
7. Salmonella
8. *Mycobact. tuberculosis*

CAUSES OF OSTEONECROSIS (e.g. femoral head)

1. Trauma   — Fracture or dislocation
2. Infection — Osteomyelitis
               Septic arthritis
               Tuberculosis
3. Sickle-cell disease
4. Glucocorticoid therapy
5. Caisson disease (divers)
6. Gaucher's disease
7. Irradiation
8. Perthes' disease

CAUSES OF HYPERMOBILE JOINTS

1. Marfan's
2. Ehlers–Danlos
3. Osteogenesis imperfecta
4. Homocystinuria
5. Hyperlysinaemia
6. Idiopathic

CAUSES OF GENERALIZED STIFFNESS

1. *Unaccustomed exercise*
2. *Systemic infection,* e.g. influenza
3. *Arthritis,* especially
   (i)   Rheumatoid
   (ii) Polymyalgia rheumatica
   (iii) Generalized osteoarthrosis
   (iv) Ochronosis
   (v)   Haemochromatosis
   (vi) Serum sickness
4. *Neuromuscular disease*
   (i)   'Stiff man syndrome' (tonic muscle rigidity)
   (ii) Cervical spondylosis with myelopathy
   (iii) Extrapyramidal disease
         Torsion dystonia
         Hepatolenticular degeneration (Wilson's)
         Parkinsonism
   (iv) Tetanus
   (v)   McArdle's myopathy
   (vi) Myotonia
   (vii) Dermatomyositis
5. *Scleroderma*
6. *Generalized oedema*
   (i)   Anascara
   (ii) Scleroedema
   (iii) Erythroderma
7. *Hypothyroidism,* especially in cold weather
8. *Mucopolysaccharidoses*

REFLEX SYMPATHETIC DYSTROPHY (Shoulder-hand syndrome, Sudek's atrophy)

Associated conditions
1. Myocardial infarction
2. Trauma
3. Cervical spinal lesion
4. Hemiplegia
5. Brain tumour
6. Electroconvulsive therapy
7. Pulmonary lesions
8. Herpes zoster
9. Drugs, e.g. phenobarbitone, isoniazid

CAUSES OF CARPAL TUNNEL SYNDROME

1. Idiopathic
2. Pregnancy, 'pill', premenstrual

3. Myxoedema
4. Acromegaly
5. Rheumatoid arthritis (may be presenting symptom)
6. Previous scaphoid fracture
7. Intermittent trauma
8. Amyloidosis
9. End-stage renal failure

THORACIC OUTLET SYNDROMES

1. Fascial band behind scalenus anterior
2. Cervical rib
3. Elongated transverse process of C7
4. Fracture of Ist. rib or clavicle
5. Vascular disorders
6. Postural and sleep syndromes

RAYNAUD'S PHENOMENON

Paroxysmal digital ischaemia, usually accompanied by pallor and cyanosis and followed by erythema

Causes
1. *Vasoconstriction*
   (i) Raynaud's disease
   (ii) Vibrating machinery
   (iii) Drugs, e.g. β-blockers
   (iv) Toxins
        Vinyl chloride
        Ergot
        Heavy metals
        Tobacco
2. *Arterial occlusion*
   (i) Thoracic outlet syndromes (p. 189)
   (ii) Embolus, thrombosis or stenosis
   (iii) Arteriosclerosis
   (iv) Buerger's disease
   (v) Injury (Volkmann's ischaemia)
3. *'Collagen-vascular' disease*
   (i) Systemic sclerosis
   (ii) Polyarteritis
   (iii) SLE
   (iv) Rh. arthritis, Sjøgren's
4. *Increased blood agglutination*
   (i) Cold agglutinins

   (ii) Dysproteinaemias
   (iii) Polycythaemia, leukaemia, Moschcowitz's, etc.
5. *Neurological:* paralysis or disuse of a limb
6. *Cold injury:* frost bite
7. *Malnutrition and cachexia*
8. *Miscellaneous rare causes*
   Typhoid fever, amyloidosis, myxoedema, etc.

Causes of cryoglobulinaemia
1. Idiopathic
2. Collagen-vascular disease
3. Infections
   Bacterial endocarditis
   Syphilis
   Infectious mononucleosis
   Cytomegalic virus infection
   Viral hepatitis
   Leprosy
   Toxoplasmosis
4. Multiple myeloma and Waldenstrøm's macroglobulinaemia
5. Myeloproliferative disease
6. Miscellaneous
   Sickle-cell disease
   Glomerulonephritis
   Myocardial infarction
   Ulcerative colitis
   Chronic liver disease, etc.

RHEUMATOID DISEASE

ARA criteria for diagnosis of rheumatoid arthritis
1. Morning stiffness
2. Swelling of three or more joints for six weeks or more
3. Swelling of wrist, MCP or PIP joints for six weeks or more
4. Symmetrical joint swelling
5. Typical X-ray changes of RA
6. Rheumatoid nodules
7. Positive rheumatoid factor

Definite rheumatoid = 4 or more of above

Complications of rheumatoid disease
1. *Poor general health*
   (i)   Weight loss
   (ii) Anaemia
   (iii) Depression and social problems

2. *Joint complications*
   (i) Deformity, subluxation, etc.
   (ii) Pyoarthrosis
   (iii) Tendon rupture, due to attrition or nodules
   (iv) Nerve compression, due to tenosynovial swelling
   (v) Cord or root compression, due to cervical subluxation
   (vi) Baker's synovial cyst
   (vii) Acute rupture of synovial sac, especially in knee
   (viii) Hoarseness, due to cricoarytenoid arthritis
   (ix) Deafness, due to arthritis of auditory ossicles
3. *Pressure sores and infected ulcers*
4. *Osteoporosis and muscle atrophy*
5. *Pulmonary*
   (i) Pleuritis, effusion
   (ii) Nodule in lung or pleura
   (iii) Fibrosing alveolitis
   (iv) Caplan's syndrome in pneumoconiosis
6. *Cardiac*
   (i) Pericarditis
   (ii) Rheumatoid granuloma of heart
7. *Ocular*
   (i) Scleritis
   (ii) Scleromalacia perforans
   (iii) Sjøgren's syndrome
8. *Arteritis*
   (i) Digital ischaemia (may be Raynaud's)
   (ii) Leg ulcers
   (iii) Mesenteric ischaemia
   (iv) Arteritis of lungs, kidneys, liver, etc.
9. *Peripheral and autonomic neuropathy*
10. *Lymphadenopathy*
   Usually in region of an inflamed joint
11. *Amyloidosis*
   May develop renal vein thrombosis
12. *Hyperviscosity syndrome* due to macromolecule polymerization (esp. RA factor)
13. *Felty's syndrome* (Splenomegaly, RA and leukopenia)
14. *Complications of therapy*
15. *Associated auto-immune disease*
   (i) Pernicious anaemia
   (ii) Thyroiditis
   (iii) Haemolytic anaemia, etc.
16. *Subfertility* (Prior to development of arthritis)

Factors in the anaemia of RA

1. Fe deficiency
   (i) GI blood loss due to drugs (aspirin, NSAIDs, glucocorticoids)
   (ii) Defective Fe utilization ('anaemia of chronic disorders')

2. Folic acid deficiency
3. Marrow hypoplasia (including drug-induced)
4. Haemodilution
5. Haemolysis, especially in Felty's syndrome
6. Increased incidence of pernicious anaemia

Conditions in which rheumatoid factor may be present
1. Collagen-vascular disease, especially Sjøgren's syndrome and rheumatoid disease
2. Infection
   (i)   Syphilis
   (ii) Kala-azar
   (iii) Leprosy
   (iv) Infective endocarditis
   (v)   Tuberculosis
   (vi) Rubella
   (vii) Infectious mononucleosis
3. Sarcoidosis
4. Asbestosis
5. Chronic liver disease
6. Post-blood transfusion
7. Malignancy
8. Waldenstrøm's macroglobulinaemia
9. Renal transplantation
10. Glomerulonephritis
11. Relatives of RA patients
12. Normal old age

Conditions associated with Sjøgren's syndrome
1. Collagen-vascular disease
2. Hashimoto's thyroiditis
3. Peripheral neuropathy
4. Renal tubular acidosis
5. Primary biliary cirrhosis
6. Diffuse interstitial pulmonary fibrosis
7. Cryoglobulinaemia
8. Hyperglobulinaemic purpura (Waldenstrøm)
9. Lymphoma
10. Pancreatitis
11. HIV infection

LUPUS ERYTHEMATOSUS

ARA Criteria for diagnosis of SLE (1982)
1. Malar erythema
2. Discoid lupus
3. Photosensitivity

4. Oral ulceration
5. Arthritis, non-erosive, of 2 or more joints
6. Cellular casts or proteinuria (more than 500 mg/day)
7. Pleurisy or pericarditis
8. Psychosis or convulsions with no other cause
9. Haemolytic anaemia, leukopenia, lymphopenia or thrombocytopenia
10. Immunological: LE cells, raised anti-DNA titre, anti-Sm or false positive VDRL
11. Antinuclear antibody

The presence of four or more features strongly suggests SLE

Conditions in which antinuclear antibodies may be present
1. Collagen–vascular disease, esp. SLE
2. Chronic liver disease
3. Hashimoto's thyroiditis, thymoma, myasthenia gravis
4. Pernicious anaemia
5. Tuberculosis
6. Leprosy
7. Diffuse pulmonary fibrosis
8. Lymphoma or other malignancy
9. Ulcerative colitis
10. Normal old people

Major antinuclear and anticytoplasmic antibodies
Antigen	Antibody
DNA	Anti-double-stranded DNA Ab. is highly specific for DNA
RNA	Ab. to ribonucleotides, found in SLE and SS
RNP	Ab. to a complex antigen of RNA and protein, found in subsets of SLE
Ro(SSA)	Cytoplasmic Ab. found in Sjøgren's, ANA-negative lupus, neonatal lupus (often with congenital heart block), the mothers of such babies, and in idiopathic thrombo-cytopenic purpura
La(SSB)	Usually in association with anti-Ro Ab.
Sm	Usually in association with anti-RNP Ab., esp. in Negroes with SLE
Jo-1	Occurs in polymyositis
Histone	Antihistones occur in some drug-induced lupus, e.g. procaineamide
SCL-70	Systemic sclerosis
ANCA	Necrotizing vasculitis

Conditions associated with antineutrophilic cytoplasmic antibodies (ANCAs)
1. Wegener's granulomatosis
2. Microscopic polyarteritis
3. Churg–Strauss syndrome

4. SLE
5. Atrial myxoma
6. HIV infection
7. Rheumatoid arthritis

c-ANCA (cytoplasmic pattern) is more specific for Wegener's than p-ANCA (perinuclear)

Rheumatic conditions associated with HIV infection
1. Reactive arthritis
2. Arthralgia
3. Psoriatic arthritis
4. Polymyositis
5. Sjøgren's syndrome
6. Necrotizing vasculitis
7. Septic arthritis

NECROTIZING VASCULITIS

No classification is completely satisfactory, since the clinical syndromes may overlap, and their pathogenesis is imperfectly understood
1. *Polyarteritis nodosa*
     (i)   Classical systemic
     (ii) Cutaneous
2. *Giant cell arteritis*
     (i)   Cranial arteritis
     (ii) Polymyalgia rheumatica
     (iii) Aortic arch syndrome (including Takayasu's)
3. *Granulomatous*
     (i)   Wegener's granuloma and lethal midline granuloma
     (ii) Allergic granulomatosis (Churg)
     (iii) Lymphomatoid granulomatosis
4. *Rheumatic and collagen diseases*
     (i)   Rheumatoid
     (ii) SLE
     (iii) Dermatomyositis
     (iv) Systemic sclerosis
     (v)   Rheumatic fever
5. *Leukocytoclastic* (neutrophilic infiltrate with nuclear fragmentation)
     (i)   Leukocytoclastic vasculitis (Zeek)
     (ii) Henoch–Schönlein purpura
     (iii) Hypocomplementaemic vasculitis (often urticarial)
     (iv) Essential mixed cryoglobulinaemia
     (v)   Hyperglobulinaemic purpura (Waldenström)

(vi)   Erythema nodosum, nodular vasculitis or erythema
       induration
(vii) Erythema elevatum diutinum
6. *Infective*
   (i)   Extension of perivascular inflammation, e.g. cellulitis,
         abscess
   (ii) Septicaemia, septic emboli
   (iii) Cutaneous arteritis during rash of meningococcaemia,
         scarlatina, typhus fever, etc.

Dermatology

SKIN CHANGES ASSOCIATED WITH SYSTEMIC MALIGNANCY

A. Genetic syndromes predisposing to neoplasm
1. *Phakomatoses* (disseminated hamartomata of eye, skin and brain)
   - (i) Neurofibromatosis (von Recklinghausen's)
   - (ii) Epiloia (Bourneville's, tuberous sclerosis)
   - (iii) Basal cell naevoid syndrome (Gorlin's)
   - (iv) Cerebellar haemangioblastoma (von Hippel–Lindau)
   - (v) Encephalotrigeminal angiomatosis (Sturge–Weber's)
2. *Familial tylosis* (keratoderma) and Ca. oesophagus
3. *Familial polyposis coli* (Gardner's) with sebaceous cysts
4. *Defective immunosurveillance*
   - (i) Wiskott–Aldrich
   - (ii) Ataxia telangiectasia
   - (iii) Chediak–Higashi
5. *Small intestinal polyposis* with perioral lentigines (Peutz–Jegher's syndrome). Rarely associated with carcinoma
6. *Multiple endocrine adenomatosis* (Type 2b) with pigmentation, mucosal neuromas and medullary Ca. thyroid
7. *Werner's* premature ageing syndrome
8. *Cowden's disease*. Tricholemmomata on face, oral mucosa and hands antedating Ca. of breast, thyroid or female reproductive tract
9. *Torre's syndrome*. Sebaceous adenoma or carcinoma with internal malignancy

B. Signs of exposure to a carcinogen
1. Cutaneous signs of AIDS (p. 213)
2. Nicotine staining of fingers
3. Signs of arsenic ingestion
   - (i) Keratoses
   - (ii) Diffuse pigmentation with 'rain-drops' of paler normal skin
4. Bowen's disease of covered skin
5. X-ray dermatitis or multiple basal cell ca. over spine may indicate increased risk of leukaemia

C. Direct involvement of skin by malignancy
1. Direct spread, e.g. carcinoma erysipeloides or carcinoma telangiectoides
2. Metastases
3. Paget's disease of skin (nipple or perineum)
4. Leukaemic infiltrate
5. Skin changes of lymphoma
   (i)   Prelymphomatous poikiloderma
   (ii) Cutaneous spread of a systemic lymphoma
   (iii) Mycosis fungoides and Sézary's syndrome

D. Hormone effects
1. Tumours of endocrine tissue
   Pituitary, adrenal, ovary or testis
   Note also necrolytic migratory erythema due to pancreatic glucagonoma
2. Tumours of non-endocrine tissue
   Ectopic ACTH, carcinoid, erythropoietin etc. (p. 157)

E. Other associations
1. Pigmentation
2. Pallor
3. Pruritus (esp. lymphoma)
4. Acanthosis nigricans and papillomatosis (esp. GI malignancy)
5. Dermatomyositis
6. Hypertrophic pulmonary osteoarthropathy
7. Herpes zoster (esp. lymphoma)
8. Acquired ichthyosis (esp. lymphoma)
9. Figurate erythema, e.g. Erythema gyratum repens
10. Rapid onset of multiple basal-cell papillomata (Leser–Trélat)
11. Hypertrichosis lanuginosa (acquired)
12. Widespread viral infection (eczema herpeticum, etc.) due to immune paresis of malignancy
13. Lymphoedema due to lymphatic obstruction by malignancy
14. Generalized hyperhidrosis
15. Nodular panniculitis (esp. Ca. pancreas)
16. Superficial migratory thrombophebitis (esp. Ca. pancreas)
17. Bullous pyoderma of leukaemia
18. Bullous eruptions, e.g. pemphigoid in choriocarcinoma

Acanthosis nigricans
Classification
1. Hereditary benign (irregular dominant gene)
2. Malignant acanthosis nigricans
   Usually adenocarcinoma of GI tract
3. Benign
   Associated with numerous metabolic diseases which have increased insulin resistance: (*contd*)

   e.g. obesity, acromegaly, polycystic ovaries, hypogonadal
   syndromes (Prader–Willi, Alstrom), diabetes mellitus, etc.
HAIR-AN syndrome refers to females with Hyper-androgenism,
Insulin Resistance, Acanthosis Nigricans
   4. Drug-induced
      (a) Hormones, esp. oestrogens
      (b) Nicotinic acid
      (c) Triazinate

FLUSHING

Causes of facial flushing
   1. *Alcohol*
      (i) Marked racial variation (severe in Mongoloids)
      (ii) Severe after disulfiram
      (iii) Chlorpropamide (in non-insulin-dependent diabetes)
      (iv) Inhalation of industrial solvents ('degreasers' flush')
   2. *Menopause*
      Associated with pulsatile release of luteinizing hormone, and
      presumed disturbance of hypothalamic thermoregulatory centre
   3. *Rosacea*
      May be exaggeration of normal 'heat response'
   4. *Food and drugs*
      (i) 'Dumping' syndrome
      (ii) Monosodium glutamate ('Chinese restaurant' syndrome)
      (iii) Capsaicin in peppers
      (iv) Nitrites in cured meats, and in 'recreational' drugs
      (v) Morphine injection
      (vi) Nicotinic acid
      (vii) Calcium-channel blockers
      (viii) TRH injection
   5. *Neoplasia*
      (i) Carcinoid syndrome
      (ii) Systemic mastocytosis
      (iii) Medullary Ca thyroid
      (iv) Pancreatic tumours
   6. *Neurological*
      (i) CNS   a. psychological, e.g. blush, anxiety
               b. organic lesions, e.g. Parkinsonism
      (ii) Auriculotemporal syndrome (gustatory sweating)
      (iii) Autonomic hyperreflexia

SCLERODERMA

Scleroderma refers to sclerosis (induration) of the skin and
subcutaneous tissue, but some authorities restrict the term to
morphoea and systemic sclerosis, and use the term
pseudoscleroderma for sclerosis due to other causes

Causes of scleroderma

1. *Immune*
   Systemic sclerosis or morphoea
   Mixed connective tissue disease
   Eosinophilic fasciitis
   Dermatomyositis
   SLE
   Rheumatoid disease
   Graft versus host disease
2. *Tumours*
   Carcinoid
3. *Metabolic*
   Cutaneous porphyria
   Amyloidosis
   Chronic scurvy (esp. legs)
   Mucinous infiltrate, e.g. scleroedema of Buschke, lichen
      myxoedematosus
4. *Genetic*
   Werner's progeria
5. *Drugs and toxins*
   Bleomycin, pentazocine, silica, vinyl chloride
6. *Others*
   Gravitational oedema (chronic, severe)

PORPHYRIA

Simplified synthetic pathway of haem

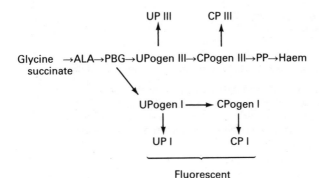

Key: ALA = amino-laevulinic acid
   PBG = porphobilinogen
   UP   = uroporphyrin
   CP   = corproporphyrin
   PP   = protoporphyrin

A specific enzyme defect has now been established in every form of porphyria

HEPATIC PORPHYRIAS

A. Genetic autosomal dominant
1. *Acute intermittent porphyria (AIP)*
Classical triad of dark urine, abdominal pain and neuropsychiatric symptoms. May be nausea, constipation, tachycardia, electrolyte disturbances and pigmentation but *no* frank photosensitivity. Acute attacks precipitated by drugs (barbiturates, sulphonamides, choloroquine, oestrogen and griseofulvin)
Lab.
  (i)   Urine darkens on standing and may fluoresce pink under UV radiation
  (ii) Watson–Schwartz Test +ve
        2 ml urine + 2 ml Ehrlich's aldehyde reagent + 4 ml saturated sodium acetate soln. A purple colour is due to *porphobilinogen* or urobilinogen, but urobilinogen is soluble in chloroform
  (iii) Urinary ALA and PBG are markedly increased, but porphyrins are normal or only slightly increased

2. *Porphyria variegata*
   Clinical features of both AIP and PCT
3. *Chester porphyria*
   Features of AIP and variegate porphyria, with psychosis, hypertension and renal disease
4. *Hereditary coproporphyria*
   Rare, resembles AIP

B. Porphyria cutanea tarda (PCT)
Photosensitivity, skin fragility, pigmentation and hirsutism

The genetic enzyme defect (hepatic uroporphyrinogen decarboxylase) is probably expressed only when the liver is damaged, particularly by iron. Most patients are middle-aged alcoholics, but hexachlorobenzene poisoning and hepatic neoplasm can also cause PCT

Lab.
  (i)   Urine fluoresces pink, due to increased UP III and CP III
  (ii) Faecal CP III increased
  (iii) Raised Se iron

ERYTHROPOIETIC PORPHYRIAS

1. Congenital erythropoietic porphyria (Gunther's disease)
Very rare defect in haem synthesis characterized by pink teeth, hypertrichosis and severe photosensitivity leading to mutilating ulceration. May be haemolytic anaemia and splenomegaly

2. Erythrohepatic protoporphyria
(Formerly called erythropoietic protoporphyria)
A familial syndrome with a variety of photosensitivity changes, burning pain characteristically relieved by cold running water, superficial linear scars (pseudorhagades) and a high incidence of gallstones.

Lab.
    (i) Erythrocyte PP is invariably increased
   (ii) Urinary porphyrins normal

Diagnosis of the porphyrias
Remember that:
1. In an acute porphyric attack, the fresh urine may be normal colour and non-fluorescent
2. Urine tests are unreliable for the detection of cutaneous porphyrias, and examination of blood and faeces is necessary

CAUSES OF PHOTOSENSITIVITY
1. *Circulating photosensitizers*
    (i) Porphyrins
   (ii) Drugs
          Amiodarone
          Psoralens
          Phenothiazines
          Diuretics
          Oral antidiabetics
          Tetracyclines (esp. demethylchlortetracycline)
          Nalidixic acid
          Sulphonamides
          Benoxaprofen (now withdrawn)
2. *Contact photosensitizers*
    (i) Tar products
   (ii) Furocoumarins (perfumes and plants)
  (iii) Chemicals in soaps and bleaches
3. *Idiopathic dermatoses*
    (i) Photosensitive eczema and actinic reticuloid
        sometimes called chronic actinic dermatitis, associated with plant allergy, esp. *Compositae* family
   (ii) Polymorphic light eruption

    (iii) Hydroa vacciniforme
    (iv) Solar urticaria
4. *Lack of protection from UVR* (decreased melanin in skin)
    (i) Albinism and vitiligo
    (ii) Phenylketonuria
    (iii) Hypopituitarism
5. *Metabolic defect*
    (i) Pellagra
    (ii) Hartnup disease
6. *Rare congenital diseases*
    e.g. Xeroderma pigmentosum, poikiloderma congenitale, etc.

UVR may also precipitate or exacerbate other dermatoses such as LE, herpes simplex and rosacea

PIGMENTATION

CAUSES OF DIFFUSE HYPERPIGMENTATION

1. *Congenital*
    (i) Racial or genetic
    (ii) Fanconi's syndrome (pancytopenia with multiple congenital defects)
2. *Physical agents*
    (i) Radiation, e.g. UVR
    (ii) Chronic rubbing, e.g. 'vagabond's itch'
3. *Post-inflammatory,* e.g. erythroderma
4. *Endocrine*
    (i) Pregnancy, oral contraceptives
    (ii) Hypoadrenalism
    (iii) Acromegaly
    (iv) Hyperthyroidism
    (v) Phaeochromocytoma
    (vi) ACTH therapy or ectopic ACTH from carcinoma
5. *Cachexia of any cause* (esp. malignancy)
6. *Chronic infection*
    Especially malaria, kala-azar, TB, bacterial endocarditis, AIDS
7. *Nutritional deficiency*
    (i) Malabsorption (esp. sprue)
    (ii) Isolated A, C, B_{12} or folate deficiency
    (iii) Pellagra
8. *Hepatic disease* (esp. biliary cirrhosis, haemochromatosis and hepatolenticular degeneration)
9. *Chronic renal failure due to increased MSH*
10. *Collagen-vascular disease*
    (i) Systemic sclerosis
    (ii) Juvenile RA (Still's)
    (iii) Dermatomyositis
    (iv) SLE

11. *Cutaneous porphyria*
12. *Drugs and chemicals*
    (i) Arsenicals
    (ii) Amiodarone
    (iii) Minocycline
    (iv) Busulphan
    (v) ACTH
    (vi) Oestrogens
    (vii) Chlorpromazine
    (viii) Chloroquine
    (ix) Photodynamic agents, e.g. psoralens
13. *Pigmentation not due to melanin*
    (i) Jaundice—yellow
    (ii) Carotenaemia—yellow
    (iii) Mepacrine—yellow
    (iv) Ochronosis (alkaptanuria)—blue-black
    (v) Argyria (due to silver)—slate-grey
    (vi) Chrysiasis (due to gold)—blue-grey
    (vii) Haemosiderosis (due to iron)—red-brown

CAUSES OF HYPOMELANOSIS (MELANIN DEFICIENCY)

A. Circumscribed depigmented patches

Congenital
1. Piebaldism (partial albinism)
2. Waardenburg's syndrome (characteristic facies, with deafness and a white forelock)
3. Tuberous sclerosis (epiloia)
4. Naevus depigmentosus

Acquired
1. Post-inflammatory
    (i) Pityriasis alba
    (ii) Eczema, esp. in Negro
    (iii) Discoid lupus erythematosus
    (iv) Scarring, e.g. burns, varicella
2. Infection
    (i) Pityriasis versicolor
    (ii) Pinta
    (iii) Leprosy
3. Immunological
    (i) Vitiligo
    (ii) Halo naevus (with circulating antimelanoma antibody)
    (iii) Malignant melanoma
4. Toxins
    (i) Hydroquinones
    (ii) Phenolic germicides

B. Generalized diffuse hypomelanosis

Congenital
1. Albinism
2. Phenylketonuria
3. Chediak—Higashi syndrome (with defective leukocytes and platelets)

Acquired
Hypopituitarism

Conditions associated with vitiligo
1. Organ-specific autoimmune disease
    (i)   Thyroiditis
    (ii) Adrenalitis
    (iii) Pernicious anaemia
    (iv) Juvenile-onset diabetes mellitus
2. Alopecia areata
3. Morphea
4. Halo naevus (Sutton's naevus)
5. Malignant melanoma
6. Sunburn and skin cancer

HIRSUTISM

Growth in the female of coarse terminal hair in the male adult
sexual pattern

CAUSES

1. Idiopathic
A heterogenous group which includes racial and familial variation.
In some cases there is excessive androgen production, usually
ovarian, but sometimes adrenal. Obesity and insulin resistance may
be important

2. Ovarian disease
   (i)   Polycystic ovaries
         The full Stein–Leventhal syndrome (obesity, amenorrhoea,
         sterility, polycystic ovaries but no virilization) is relatively
         rare, but partial forms are much commoner
   (ii) Postmenopausal ovarian stromal hyperplasia
   (iii) Ovarian hilus-cell hyperplasia
   (iv) Ovarian virilizing tumours, e.g. androblastoma
   (v)   Gonadal dysgenesis

3. **Adrenal disease**
   - (i)   ACTH-dependent cortical hyperplasia
       Cushing's
       Ectopic ACTH syndrome
   - (ii) Adrenal tumours
   - (iii) Late-onset congenital adrenal hyperplasia (C21 or
       11β-hydroxylase defect)

4. **Androgenic drugs**
Anabolic steroids
Progestogens

HYPERTRICHOSIS

Excessive hair growth in any site

Causes of generalized hypertrichosis
1. Cachexia, especially in children
2. Hereditary diseases
   e.g. erythrohepatic porphyria
       epidermolysis bullosa
       Cornelia de Lange syndrome
       trisomy E
       Hurler's syndrome
3. Head injury, especially in children
4. Dermatomyositis
5. Drugs
   - (i)   Cyclosporin A
   - (ii) Minoxidil
   - (iii) Diazoxide
   - (iv) Phenytoin
6. Hypertrichosis lanuginosa
   This may be congenital or secondary to internal malignancy

CAUSES OF ALOPECIA

1. Male-pattern baldness
2. Idiopathic diffuse alopecia of women—usually post-menopausal
3. 'Telogen effluvium'—loss of club hairs after febrile illness,
   surgery or parturition
4. Alopecia areata
5. Drugs:
   - (i)   Cytotoxic agents
   - (ii) Anticoagulants
   - (iii) Dextran
   - (iv) Oral contraceptives
6. Scalp infection:
   - (i)   Fungi
   - (ii) Pyogenic bacteria

7. Systemic disease:
   (i) Syphilis
   (ii) AIDS
   (iii) Hypothyroidism
   (iv) Fe deficiency
8. Traumatic:
   (i) Traction from rollers
   (ii) Scalping injury
   (iii) Burns
   (iv) Excessive bleaching, perming, etc.
9. Dermatoses:
   (i) Psoriasis
   (ii) Discoid lupus erythematosus
   (iii) Lichen planus
10. Congenital—many rare diseases, e.g. monilethrix

NAIL CHANGES IN SYSTEMIC DISEASE

1. Clubbing (p. 39)
2. Flat nail plate
   Cirrhosis
3. Koilonychia
   (i) Fe deficiency anaemia
   (ii) Haemochromatosis
   (iii) Thyrotoxicosis
4. Beau's lines
   (i) Acute serious or febrile illness
   (ii) Acute hypocalcaemia
5. Onycholysis
   (i) Thyrotoxicosis
   (ii) Systemic sclerosis
6. Pale nails
   Anaemia
7. Pale nails with reddish-brown distal zone ('half and half nails')
   Chronic renal failure
8. Opaque white nails, often with distal pink zone (Terry's nails)
   Cirrhosis
9. Paired narrow white transverse bands (Muehrke's lines)
   Hypoalbuminaemia
10. Transverse white line
    Hodgkin's disease
11. Red nails
    (i) Polycythaemia (reddish-blue)
    (ii) Carbon monoxide poisoning (cherry-red)
12. Red lunulae
    Cardiac failure

13. Blue nails
    (i) Cyanosis
    (ii) Wilson's hepatolenticular degeneration (azure)
    (iii) Ochronosis (slaty)
14. Yellow nail (slow growing, thick and excessively curved)
    Yellow nail syndrome with lymphoedema and pulmonary
    disease (bronchitis, bronchiectasis, effusion)
15. Splinter haemorrhages
    (i) Subacute bact. endocarditis
    (ii) Vasculitis, esp. rheumatoid disease, SLE, Behçet's
    (iii) Indwelling arterial catheter
    (iv) Trichiniasis in larval stage
    (v) Chronic mountain sickness (Monge)
    (vi) AIDS
    (vii) Cryoglobulinaemia?
NB Trauma is the commonest cause
16. Brittle nails with splitting and flaking
    (i) Digital ischaemia, esp. Raynaud's
    (ii) Myxoedema
    (iii) Chronic hypocalcaemia
    (iv) Systemic amyloidosis
    (v) Glucagonoma
17. Thick irregular cuticles
    Dermatomyositis
18. Nail-fold erythema and telangiectasia
    SLE, systemic sclerosis or dermatomyositis
19. Periungual fibroma (Koenen's tumour)
    Tuberous sclerosis
20. Many nail changes can be caused by drugs, e.g. brown
    pigment due to cytotoxics, photo-onycholysis due to tetracycline

CAUSES OF LEG ULCERS

1. Venous hypertension
   Pathogenesis may relate to pericapillary fibrin cuff, capillary
   stasis, neutrophil aggregates or depletion of growth factors
2. Ischaemia
   (i) Atheroma
   (ii) Arteritis (e.g. cutaneous polyarteritis, SLE)
   (iii) Microthrombi, e.g. due to anticardiolipin antibody
3. Lymphatic obstruction
   (i) Congenital (Milroy's disease)
   (ii) Acquired, e.g. filariasis
4. Neuropathy
   (i) Diabetes mellitus
   (ii) Spina bifida
   (iii) Tabes dorsalis
   (iv) Leprosy (in endemic areas)

5. Panniculitis
6. Trauma, esp. in thin skin due to steroid therapy
7. Infection, esp. severe erysipelas or deep mycosis
8. Malignancy—usually squamous-cell carcinoma
9. Haemolytic anaemia, especially sickle-cell
10. Necrobiosis lipoidica (may be diabetic)
11. Pyoderma gangrenosum
12. Systemic hypertension (rare)
13. Gumma is now *very* rare in UK

Many leg ulcers have a multifactorial aetiology, e.g. ischaemia, immobility, anaemia, venous hypertension and infection. This applies especially to the elderly and to rheumatoid patients

CAUSES OF BLISTERS

1. Physical
     (i)   Friction
     (ii) Burns
     (iii) Sunburn
     (iv) Prolonged pressure, especially in coma due to barbiturate overdose
2. Infection or infestation
     (i)   Viral, e.g. herpes simplex or herpes zoster/varicella
     (ii) Bacterial, e.g. bullous impetigo or erysipelas
     (iii) Scabies
3. Insect bites or stings
     e.g. due to horse flies or mosquitoes (especially in 'allergic' subjects)
4. Eczema (q.v.)
5. Immunological
     (i)   Erythema multiforme
     (ii) Dermatitis herpetiformis
     (iii) Pemphigoid
     (iv) Pemphigus
     (v)   Cutaneous vasculitis (usually haemorrhagic)
     (vi) SLE or lichen planus (rare)
6. Metabolic
     (i)   Porphyria cutanea tarda
     (ii) High doses of frusemide in renal failure
     (iii) Diabetes mellitus (rare)
7. Drug reactions
     Especially photosensitivity, e.g. due to nalidixic acid
8. Congenital
     (i)   Epidermolysis bullosa
           Many types, e.g. simple (intraepidermal split)
                              junctional (lamina lucida split)
                              dystrophic (sublamina densa split)

(ii)   Ichthyosiform erythroderma
(iii)   Incontinentia pigmenti
(iv)   Urticaria pigmentosa (after rubbing)

ECZEMA (now used as a synonym for dermatitis)

An inflammatory response of the skin characterized clinically by itching, clustered papulovesicles with erythema and scaling, and histologically by spongiosis (epidermal oedema)

Common types of eczema

A. *Exogenous*
1. Contact dermatitis
    (i)   Primary irritant, e.g. solvents, detergents, caustics, industrial coolants, etc.
          A primary irritant will cause dermatitis in a normal subject if applied in a high concentration for a prolonged period
    (ii)   Allergy, e.g. to nickel, rubber, medicaments, etc.
          An allergen will not cause dermatitis in a normal subject, although some potent allergens will rapidly induce hypersensitivity
2. Infective dermatitis
    e.g. around an infected wound or fungal infection

B. *Endogenous*
1. Atopic eczema (infantile eczema)
2. Discoid (nummular) eczema
3. Seborrhoeic dermatitis
4. Asteatotic eczema
    Due to excessive drying of the skin
5. Gravitational eczema
    Secondary to venous hypertension
6. Pompholyx
    Blisters on the palms or soles. May be endogenous or exogenous

CUTANEOUS EFFECTS OF DRUGS

1. *Exanthemata* (scarlatiniform, morbilliform, papular, etc.)
   Barbiturates, antibiotics, chloral hydrate, etc.
2. *Urticaria*
   Penicillin, salicylates, etc.
3. *Exfoliative dermatitis* (erythroderma)
   Barbiturates, arsenicals, heavy metals, etc.
4. *Fixed eruptions*
   Barbiturates, sulphonamides, phenolphthalein
5. *Bullous eruptions*
    (i)   Bromides, iodides, barbiturates, etc.

    (ii)   Erythema multiforme (including Stevens–Johnson syndrome) and toxic epidermal necrolysis: Sulphonamides, barbiturates, etc.

    (iii) Pemphigus: Penicillamine

6. *Purpura*
   - (i)   Drugs causing aplastic anaemia (p. 81)
   - (ii) Selective thrombocytopenia: Sedormid, quinine
   - (iii) Vascular: carbromal, glucocorticoids, penicillin, etc.

7. *Photosensitivity* (toxicity or allergy) (p. 201)

8. *Erythema nodosum*
   Sulphonamides

9. *Acneiform*
   Glucocorticoids, androgens, iodides, bromides, INAH, anticonvulsants, cyanocobalamin, lithium

10. *Lichenoid*
    Antimalarials, chlorothiazide, amiphenazole, gold

11. *Pigmentation* (p. 203)

12. *Hypertrichosis or hirsutism* (p. 204)

13. *Hair loss*
    Cytotoxics, anticoagulants, retinoids

14. *Ichthyosis*
    Nicotinic acid, triparanol

15. *Eczema*
    Systemic administration of a drug after allergic contact dermatitis to the drug has developed

16. *Seborrhoeic dermatitis*
    Methyldopa

17. *SLE-like syndrome*
    Procainamide, hydrallazine, hydantoins, sulphonamides, etc.

18. *Psoriasiform*
    β-blockers, esp. practolol (now withdrawn)

19. *Scleroderma* (p. 199)

20. *Nail pigmentation*
    Cytotoxics, esp. busulphan

21. *Palmoplantar desquamation*
    Retinoids

22. *Cheilitis and nasal crusting*
    Retinoids

23. *Flushing* (p. 198)

24. *Cutis laxa, morphoea or elastoma perforans*
    Penicillamine

25. *Livedo reticularis*
    Amantadine

26. *Exacerbation of pre-existing skin disease*
    Porphyria—sulphonamides, barbiturates, chloroquine, oestrogens, griseofulvin
    Psoriasis—chloroquine, lithium

PRURITUS

Systemic causes of generalized pruritus
1. *Hepatic*
   Obstructive jaundice
   Recurrent pruritus of pregnancy
2. *Chronic renal failure* (may be due to secondary hyperparathyroidism)
3. *Blood*
   AIDS
   Malignant lymphoma
   Myeloproliferative disorders
   Fe-deficiency
   Mastocytosis
4. *Carcinoma,* especially lung, stomach, colon, breast
5. *Endocrine*
   Myxoedema or hyperthyroidism
   Carcinoid
6. *Drugs*
   Cocaine, morphine, stilbamidine
   Allergic drug reactions
7. *Parasites:* roundworm, trichiniasis, onchocerciasis, etc.
8. *Neurological*
   Tabes or GPI
   Multiple sclerosis
9. *Psychogenic*

Causes of severe pruritus due to skin disease
1. Mites (including scabies), insect bites, pediculosis
2. Eczema
3. Urticaria
4. Lichen planus
5. Dermatitis herpetiformis
6. Lichen simplex chronicus
7. Miliaria rubra (prickly heat)

Causes of palmar erythema
1. Dermatoses, e.g. eczema, tinea, psoriasis, pityriasis rubra pilaris
2. Increased oestrogens
   (i) Pregnancy
   (ii) Cirrhosis, especially alcoholic
3. Arthritis, especially rheumatoid
4. Shoulder-hand syndrome
5. Polycythaemia
6. Beri-beri
7. Mitral insufficiency
8. Diabetes mellitus

Dermatoses which exhibit the Köbner phenomenon
(development of lesions at site of skin trauma)
1. Psoriasis
2. Lichen planus
3. Eczema
4. Keloids
5. Sarcoidosis
6. Viral warts
7. Vitiligo

MALIGNANT MELANOMA

Features of value in clinical identification

A. Major
1. Increase in size (though growth is common during puberty or pregnancy)
2. Change in shape, or irregular margin
3. Change in colour, or irregularity of pigmentation

B. Minor
1. Diameter more than 7 mm
2. Inflammation
3. Bleeding or oozing
4. Itch

Prognosis for excised melanoma depends on *Breslow thickness* (vertical height from granular layer to deepest identifiable malignant cell)

	5–year survival
Less than 0.76 mm—	almost 100%
0.76 to 1.5 mm—	over 80%
1.6 to 3.4 mm—	40 to 80%
More than 3.4 mm—	less than 40%

Common causes of a pigmented papule
1. Basal cell papilloma ('seborrhoeic wart')
2. Melanocytic naevus ('mole')
3. Malignant melanoma
4. Pigmented basal cell carcinoma
5. Dermatofibroma

INDUSTRIAL SKIN DISEASES

1. **Contact dermatitis**
   (i) Due to irritants
       e.g. cutting oils
            caustics
            organic solvents

detergents
fibreglass
physical factors, etc.
(ii)   Due to allergies
e.g. chromate in cement, anti-rust paint, leather, etc.
cobalt in cutting tools, polyester paints, etc.
nickel in coins, jewellery, cleansing fluids, etc.
epoxy resins in plastics, electrical components, etc.
rubber chemicals (vulcanizers, accelerants and
antioxidants) in tyres, hoses, couplings, etc.
2. **Leukoderma (depigmentation)**
Due to hydroquinone derivatives, e.g. in adhesives
3. **Industrial acne**
(i)   Folliculitis due to mineral oils
(ii)   Chloracne due to halogenated hydrocarbons, e.g. dioxin
4. **Skin cancer**
Due to chronic exposure to tar, mineral oils or chloroprene
5. **Scleroderma**
Vinyl chloride disease (also causes Raynaud's, pulmonary
fibrosis, acro-osteolysis and hepatic angiosarcoma)
6. **Porphyria cutanea tarda**
Due to dioxin
7. **Fluoride spots**
Pigmented spots due to atmospheric fluoride from aluminium
smelting
8. **Lichen planus**
Due to colour film developers
9. **Chrome ulcers**

CUTANEOUS CONDITIONS ASSOCIATED WITH AIDS

1. Transient rash at time of seroconversion
Widespread maculopapular rash. May resemble urticaria or
infectious mononucleosis
2. Skin infections (often extensive, exaggerated or exotic)
(i)   Viral: herpes simplex, zoster/varicella, molluscum
contagiosum, EB virus (oral hairy leukoplakia), warts, CMV
(ii)   Bacterial: *Staph. aureus,* mycobacteria, etc.
(iii)   Fungal: *Candida, Tinea,* pityriasis versicolor, opportunist
(esp. cryptococcosis and sporotrichosis)
(iv)   Protozoal or arthropod, e.g. scabies
3. Kaposi's sarcoma
4. Bacillary angiomatosis, probably due to infection with
Rochalimaea henselae, possibly from cats

5. Miscellaneous
  (i) Seborrhoeic dermatitis, often severe (may affect up to 80%)
  (ii) Xerosis or ichthyosis
  (iii) Psoriasis may become atypical and intractable
  (iv) Papular-pruritic eruption
  (v) Ofuji's pustular folliculitis
  (vi) Immune complex vasculitis
  (vii) Telangiectasia or petechiae
  (viii) Allergy to drugs, especially sulphonamides
  (ix) Erythroderma
  (x) Cutaneous lymphoma
  (xi) Multiple basal cell cancers
  (xii) Generalized pigmentation or nail pigmentation

NB Squamous cancer of mouth and anus is commoner in the male homosexual community, but may be unrelated to HIV infection

Venereology

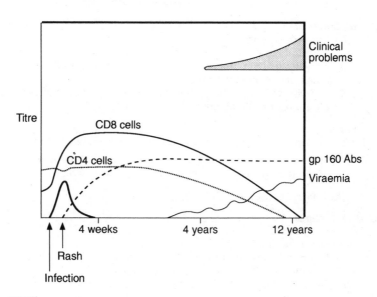

AIDS

Definition of AIDS (CDC, Atlanta, Georgia, USA): The occurrence of a
reliably diagnosed disease that is at least moderately indicative of an
underlying cellular immune deficiency (see below) in a patient with no
other known cause than HIV infection, nor any other cause of reduced
resistance reported to be associated with that disease. Patients must
have a positive test for HIV, or a low number of T helper lymphocytes

A. Infections
  1. *Viral*
      (i)   Cytomegalovirus—pulmonary, gut or CNS
      (ii) Herpes simplex virus—severe mucocutaneous disease for
            over one month; pulmonary, gut or disseminated
      (iii) Progressive multifocal leukoencephalopathy
  2. *Bacterial*
      Atypical mycobacteriosis—disseminated
  3. *Fungal*
      (i)   Candidiasis—oesophageal or bronchopulmonary
      (ii) Cryptococcus—pulmonary, CNS or disseminated
      (iii) Histoplasmosis—disseminated
      (iv) Aspergillosis—CNS or disseminated

4. *Protozoal*
   - (i) *Pneumocystis carinii* pneumonia
   - (ii) Toxoplasmosis—pneumonia or CNS
   - (iii) Cryptosporidiosis and isosporiasis—diarrhoea over I month
   - (iv) Strongyloidosis—pneumonia, CNS or disseminated

B. Malignancy
   - (i) Kaposi's sarcoma
   - (ii) Cerebral lymphoma
   - (iii) Non-Hodgkins lymphoma—diffuse, undifferentiated and of B cell or unknown phenotype
   - (iv) Lymphoreticular malignancy—more than 3 months after an opportunistic infection

C. Other
Chronic lymphoid interstitial pneumonitis in children under 13 years

The full AIDS syndrome currently occurs in only a small percentage of those infected with HIV. Two commoner syndromes are:

1. AIDS related complex (ARC)

Clinical features:
   - (i) Fatigue
   - (ii) Night sweats
   - (iii) Lymphadenopathy for 3 or more months
   - (iv) Weight loss of at least 10% body weight
   - (v) Fever for more than 3 months
   - (vi) Diarrhoea

Laboratory features:
   - (i) Low T helper cell count
   - (ii) Hyperglobulinaemia
   - (iii) Anergy to recall antigens on skin testing

ARC patients must have two clinical and two laboratory features

2. Persistent generalized lymphadenopathy (PGL)
Criteria are:
   - (i) Lymphadenopathy for 3 or more months involving at least 2 sites other than the inguinal nodes
   - (ii) Absence of any other known cause of such lymphadenopathy
   - (iii) If biopsy is performed, the node shows reactive hyperplasia

Even more patients are clinically well but HIV positive

PRESENTATION OF GONORRHOEA

1. *Primary genital infection*
   - (i) Asymptomatic 'contact'
   - (ii) Urethritis
   - (iii) Vaginitis or cervicitis

2. *Extension of infection within genital tract*
   Female: endometritis, salpingitis, cystitis, etc.
   Male: prostatitis, cystitis, epididymitis, etc.
3. *Extragenital dissemination*
   (i)   Bacteraemia, may produce rigors or may be asymptomatic
   (ii) Arthritis-dermatitis syndrome:
         Papulopustular rash
         Tenosynovitis
         Arthralgia
         Myalgia
         Pyrexia
   (iii) Mono-articular septic joint
   (iv) Endocarditis, myocarditis or pericarditis
   (v)   Hepatitis or perihepatitis
   (vi) Meningitis
   (vii) Pelvic peritonitis (in female)
4. *Primary extragenital infection*
   (i)   Conjunctivitis or ophthalmitis in neonates
   (ii) Skin infection, stomatitis, pharyngitis, proctitis, etc.
5. *Complications of the above*
   e.g. sterility after salpingitis
        stricture after urethritis

SEROLOGICAL TESTS FOR SYPHILIS

1. *Tests for reagin or antilipoidal Ab*
   Cardiolipin WR
   VDRL slide test (flocculation). May give false negatives
2. *Tests for group-reactive antitreponemal Ab*
   Reiter protein complement fixation. May give false positives
3. *Specific treponemal tests*
   (i)   Treponemal immobilization test
   (ii) *T. pallidum* immune adherence
   (iii) Fluorescent treponemal Ab test (FTA–ABS)
   (iv) *T. pallidum* haemagglutination (TPHA test)

Choice of test
1. *Early syphilis*
   (i)   *Primary.* All serology is initially negative, except FTA–ABS
         which may be positive in 80% (useful for male homosexuals)
   (ii) *Secondary.* All serology positive
2. *Late* (2 years post infection)
   Reagin tests may occasionally be negative but specific tests
   with treponemal Ag tests are positive
In practice the needs of both clinical disease and screening (e.g. blood
donors or antenatal women) can be met by a combination of tests for
reagin (VDRL) and a specific test (TPHA)

Immunology

CYTOKINES

A general term for soluble intercellular signalling molecules. They include interleukins, interferons, colony stimulating factors and tissue necrosis factors

Interleukin1. Produced by macrophages and a variety of other cells. Acts on T-cells, B-cells and macrophages. Produces many effects including fever, slow wave sleep, hypercoagulation, increased acute phase proteins, proteolysis and neutrophilia

Interleukin 2. Induces T-cell proliferation and activation both in vivo and in vitro. Also acts as a growth and differentiation factor for both B-cells and macrophages

Interleukin 3. A cytokine produced by T-cells, natural killer cells and mast cells, and which has profound effects on growth of all haemopoietic lineages

Interleukin 4. A growth factor for T-cells and may regulate B-cell differentiation

Interleukin 5. Causes eosinophil differentiation and possibly antigen production and differentiation of B-cells

Interleukin 6. Diverse actions, similar to IL-1. A major inducer of terminal differentiation of B-cells and important in synthesis of acute phase proteins by hepatocytes

Interferons. A heterogeneous group of protein mediators which increase the resistance of cells to viral infection. Subtypes IFN α, β, and γ are produced by leucocytes, fibroblasts and T-cells respectively

Tissue necrosis factor. Two cytokines, whose genes are closely linked in the MHC complex. TNFα (cachectin) is produced by macrophages, T-cells and NK cells, whereas TNFβ (lymphotoxin) is produced by activated T-cells. Act as mediators of cytotoxicity, inflammation and probably contribute to the wasting in chronic diseases

CELL SURFACE MARKERS

CD markers (clusters of differentiation). Agreed system for naming cell surface markers found on haemopoietic cells. Examples:

CD3 Pan T-cell marker, Subunit of the T-cell receptor (TCR)

CD4   MHC class II receptor, found on some T-cells (usually T helper cells)
CD8   MHC class I receptor, expressed on a mutually exclusive T-cell
      subset to CD4 and on NK cells; may show cytotoxic function
      (usually T suppressor cells)
CD25 Interleukin 2 receptor (β)
CD45 Leucocyte common antigen, three subtypes

T AND B LYMPHOCYTES

B LYMPHOCYTE DEFICIENCIES

A. Primary

Hypogammaglobulinaemia
  1. Congenital sex-linked (Bruton's)
  2. Non-sex-linked agammaglobulinaemia
  3. Hypogammaglobulinaemia of late onset
  4. Combined immunodeficiency syndromes
     (i)   Alymphocytic (Swiss-type)
     (ii) Thymic dysplasia
     (iii) Achondroplastic
Dysgammaglobulinaemia (normal γ-globulin on electrophoresis)
Types I to VII, e.g. selective deficit of IgA (Type IV) occurs in ataxia
telangiectasia, and selective deficit of IgM (Type V) in Wiskott–
Aldrich syndrome

B. Secondary
  1. *Defective synthesis*
     (i)   Prematurity or delayed maturity
     (ii) Lymphoma, myelomatosis or Waldenström's
           macroglobulinaemia
     (iii) Marrow disorders, e.g. myelosclerosis, metastases,
           hypoplasia
     (iv) Irradiation and cytotoxic drugs
  2. *Protein deficiency*
     (i)   Nephrotic syndrome
     (ii) Protein-losing enteropathy
     (iii) Severe malnutrition or malabsorption
     (iv) Exfoliative dermatitis
     (v)   Myotonic dystrophy

Causes of hypergammaglobulinaemia
  1. *Diffuse 'broad band' type* (polyclonal gammopathy)
     (i)   Chronic infection
     (ii) Hepatic disease
     (iii) 'Collagen-vascular' disease, also ulcerative colitis, Crohn's,
           Hashimoto's thyroiditis, etc.

2. *Narrow 'M band' type* (monoclonal gammopathy)
   (i) Multiple myeloma
   (ii) Waldenström's macroglobulinaemia
   (iii) 'Benign' paraproteinaemia, especially in old people
   (iv) Heavy chain disease (may be γ, μ or α)
   (v) Bence–Jones proteinuria in absence of myelomatosis
   (vi) Leukaemia, lymphoma or carcinoma
   (vii) Primary cold agglutinins
   (viii) Amyloidosis
   (ix) Lichen myxoedematosus

T LYMPHOCYTE DEFICIENCIES

A. Primary
1. Thymic and parathyroid aplasia (Di George's)
2. Lymphopenia with normal immunoglobulins (Nezelof's)
3. Episodic lymphopenia with lymphocytotoxin
4. Qualitative lymphocyte defects (e.g. chronic mucocutaneous Candidosis)

B. Secondary
1. Human immunosuppressive virus (AIDS)
2. Cytotoxic drugs
3. Malignancy, esp. T cell lymphoma
4. Various (? immunological) diseases, e.g. eczema, multiple sclerosis
5. Kwashiorkor
6. Secondary to B cell deficiency

CAUSES OF PHAGOCYTE DYSFUNCTION

1. Defective chemotaxis
   (i) Diabetes mellitus
   (ii) Steroid therapy
   (iii) Malnutrition
   (iv) Malignancy, esp. Hodgkin's disease
   (v) Renal failure
   (vi) Severe burns
   (vii) SLE and rheumatoid disease
   (viii) Granulomata (sarcoid, Crohn's)
   (ix) Some antibiotics, esp. tetracycline
   (x) Lazy leukocyte syndrome

2. Defective opsonization
   (i) Complement deficiency, e.g. C3 or C5
   (ii) IgM deficiency (e.g. in neonates)
   (iii) Sickle-cell anaemia
   (iv) Absence of spleen
   (v) SLE

3. Defective intracellular bacterial killing

(i) Chronic granulomatous disease of childhood
Lymphadenopathy, hepatomegaly, pneumonia, dermatitis, abscesses, osteomyelitis. Due to defective hydrogen peroxide production

(ii) Job's syndrome
Recurrent cold staphylococcal abscesses

(iii) Chediak–Higashi syndrome
Partial oculocutaneous albinism. Giant lysosomes in granulocytes. Recurrent bacterial infections, sometimes with a lymphomatoid reaction

(iv) Myeloperoxidase deficiency

(v) Severe glucose-6-P dehydrogenase deficiency

(vi) Drugs
Glucocorticoids, colchicine, etc.

COMPLEMENT

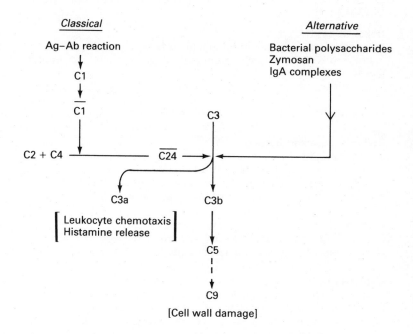

The complement cascade

The above system also interacts with the coagulation (Factor XIII) and kinin systems and there are many inhibitory and regulatory factors

Some inherited complement defects associated with clinical effects

Deficiency	Association
C1 inhibitor	Hereditary angio-oedema, due to unrestrained complement activation
C1r	SLE-like syndrome
C1s	'Immune-complex' disease
C2	Henoch-Schönlein purpura, glomerulonephritis, SLE, etc.
C3	Recurrent infections
Terminal components, C5–C9	Recurrent infections (esp. Neisseria)

CLINICAL DISEASE ASSOCIATED WITH ACQUIRED COMPLEMENT DEFICIENCY

Renal disease
In mesangiocapillary glomerulonephritis (with the C3 nephritic factor) the C3 level is low in the presence of normal C1, C2 and C4 levels
In early acute post-streptococcal glomerulonephritis, C3 and C4 are low
In SLE nephritis the C4 is often reduced more than C3

Collagen-vascular disease
In SLE the C3 and C4 are low
In active rheumatoid disease, complement levels may be increased
In polyarteritis nodosa, cranial cell arteritis and Wegener's granulomatosis the complement levels are normal

Liver disease
In acute hepatitis, C3 and C4 are low in the first week, and in chronic hepatitis the C3 may remain low

Miscellaneous
In cryoglobulinaemia, C4 is low, often with normal C3
In lymphoproliferative disease, C1 inhibitor may be deficient
In haemolytic anaemia, septicaemia, severe malaria and disseminated intravascular coagulation, C3 may be low

Skin testing for immunological reactions

Type I (immediate hypersensitivity) (*Prick test*). An urticarial wheal, developing within 20 minutes and resolving within 2 hours

Type III (circulating immune complex) (*ID injection*). An ill-defined red swelling, sometimes purpuric, developing over several hours, maximal at 5–7 hours and resolving in 24–36 hours

Type IV (delayed hypersensitivity) (*ID injection or Patch test*). An indurated red area, sometimes with vesiculation, developing within 24–48 hours and resolving over several days

BIOSYNTHESIS OF PROSTANOIDS

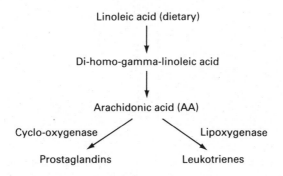

The cyclo-oxygenase pathway

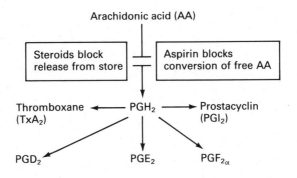

The lipoxygenase pathway

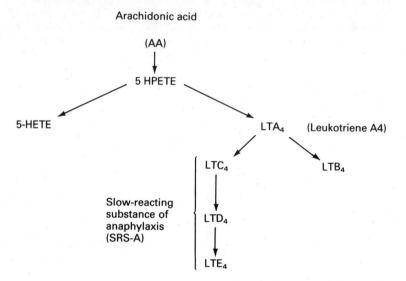

LTB$_4$ and 5-HETE stimulate neutrophil and eosinophil chemotaxis
SRS-A causes bronchiolar spasm and increased mucus secretion

Genetics and molecular biology

GLOSSARY OF TERMS

Alleles. Alternative forms of a gene at a given locus. A child should receive one of each pair of alleles from each parent

Amplification. Production of multiple copies of a DNA sequence

Aneuploid. A chromosome number which is not an exact multiple of the haploid number (q.v.) e.g. trisomy

Annealing. The coming together of complementary single-stranded nucleic acids (opposite of denaturing)

Autoradiography. A technique to detect radioactively labelled molecules as an image on a photographic emulsion

Autosome. Any chromosome other than the sex chromosomes. Man has 22 pairs of autosomes

Bacteriophage. Bacterial virus, often used as a vector (q.v.) in cloning

Barr body. The sex chromatin seen in somatic cells of the female.

Base pair (b.p.). In double-stranded DNA there is complementary purine–pyrimidine hydrogen bonding [adenosine (A) must pair with thymine (T) and guanine (G) with cytosine (C)]. Each hydrogen-bonded pair is called a base pair and the b.p. number indicates the length of a piece of DNA. The human genome has 3 billion b.p.

Carrier. An individual who is heterozygous for a normal gene and an abnormal gene which is not expressed phenotypically

Chimera. An individual composed of cells from different zygotes. In 'blood-group' chimerism dizygotic twins exchange haemopoietic stem cells in utero and continue to form blood cells of both types. In 'whole-body' chimerism two separate zygotes are fused into one individual

Chromatid. A chromosome consists of two parallel strands (chromatids) held together by the centromere

Clone. A group of genetically identical cells derived by mitosis from a single ancestral cell

Cloning vectors. Plasmids into which foreign DNA may be inserted for the purpose of cloning DNA of interest

Codon. A triplet of 3 bases in a DNA or RNA molecule specifying a single amino acid

Complementarity. Specific base pairing of nucleotide bases in nucleic acids (e.g. A to T, G to C)

Complementary DNA (cDNA). Single-stranded DNA synthesized from a specific mRNA template, using reverse transcriptase

Concordant. A term used to describe a pair of twins in which both members exhibit a certain trait

Cosmid vector. A vector (q.v.) designed to propagate very large sequences of DNA (e.g. for genomic libraries or genes with many introns)

Crossover. Exchange of genetic material between members of a chromosome pair

Deletion. A chromosomal aberration in which part of a chromosome is lost

Denaturation of nucleic acids. This refers to their conversion from double-stranded into single-stranded forms, usually by heating or chemical action (opposite of annealing)

Deoxyribonucleic acid (DNA). The polymer of which eukaryotic cell genes are composed

Diploid. The number of chromosomes in somatic cells (which is double that of the gametes). In man this is 46

Discordant. A term used to describe a pair of twins in which one shows a certain trait and the other does not

Dizygotic. Twins produced by two ova, separately fertilized

DNA polymerase. The enzyme responsible for replication of DNA. Each complementary strand of the DNA double helix is used as a template for the synthesis of a new strand

DNA rearrangements. Recombination of DNA segments

Domain. A region of the DNA sequence of a protein that can be equated with a particular function, or the corresponding section of a gene

Dot blotting. In this process DNA or RNA is extracted from cells and dotted onto nitrocellulose filters. A specific labelled probe is then added and hybridization is visualized by a technique such as autoradiography. The result is a dot-blot

Duplication. A chromosomal aberration in which part of a chromosome is duplicated

Ecogenetic disorder. A disorder resulting from an environmental factor interacting with a specific genetic factor, e.g. emphysema resulting from cigarette smoking in a patient with α-1 antitrypsin deficiency

Endonuclease. An enzyme that cuts DNA at an internal site. Restriction endonucleases cut DNA at specific nucleotide sequences

Enhancer. A DNA sequence that acts to increase the transcription of a nearby gene

Eukaryotic cell. A cell characteristic of higher organisms with a complex cell nucleus surrounded by a nuclear membrane (compare prokaryotic cell, q.v.)

Exon. The transcribed regions of a gene that are present in mature mRNA and usually contain coding information (see intron)

Exonuclease. An enzyme that cuts nucleotides one at a time from the 5' or 3' ends of a polynucleotide chain

Expressivity. The nature and severity of the phenotype of a mutant allele are a reflection of its expressivity. Autosomal dominant traits often show variable expressivity

F1. The first generation progeny of a mating

Frameshift mutation. A mutation involving an insertion or a deletion that is not an exact multiple of 3 b.p. This changes the reading frame (q.v.) of the code so it will be read as gibberish until a stop codon is encountered

Gametes. Reproductive cells which unite in pairs to form a zygote

Gene. A segment of DNA coded for the synthesis of a single polypeptide

Gene flow. The gradual diffusion of genes in a population due to migration and intermarriage

Gene library. This is created from the total mRNA extracted from a given tissue and reverse transcribed into cDNA. It is then incorporated into vectors that collectively contain the cDNA sequence of all genes that are expressed in that tissue

Gene map. The placement of genes in correct linear arrangement on specific chromosome regions

Gene probe (genetic marker). A stretch of DNA that can vary in its sequence of bases from person to person, i.e. the DNA is polymorphic in that region. More than 1000 such polymorphic regions have been identified in the human genome. Sometimes a genetic marker is close enough to a defective gene to be reliably inherited with it.

Restriction enzymes cut the DNA into smaller pieces. Some people lack, in the variable 'marker' region, the particular base sequence that the enzyme recognizes. The fragments of DNA will therefore vary in length in different individuals, producing what is known as 'restriction fragment length polymorphisms' (q.v.)

Genetic code. The base triplets (codons) that specify the 20 different amino acids

Genetic marker. A locus whose alleles are readily detectable

Genome. The full set of genes of an organism

Haploid. The chromosome number of a normal gamete. In man this is 23

Haplotype. The genotype of a group of alleles from 2 or more closely linked loci on one chromosome and usually inherited as a unit, e.g. the HLA complex

Heterogeneity. A phenotype is genetically heterogeneous if it can be produced by different genetic mechanisms

Heterozygote. An individual with 2 different alleles at a given locus on a pair of homologous chromosomes

Histones. Proteins associated with DNA, rich in basic amino acids (lysine and arginine)

Holandric. The inheritance pattern of genes of a Y chromosome (i.e. transmitted to all sons but no daughters)

Homologous chromosomes. A 'matched pair' of chromosomes, one from each parent, having the same gene loci in the same order

Homozygote. An individual with 2 identical alleles at a given locus on a pair of homologous chromosomes

Housekeeping genes. Genes that encode enzymes required for basic functions present in virtually all cells

Hybridization:
(i) In molecular genetics, complementary pairing of an RNA and a DNA strand or of 2 different DNA or 2 RNA strands

(ii) In cell genetics, fusion of 2 somatic cells to form a hybrid cell containing genetic information from both parent cells

Human leukocyte antigen genes (HLA genes). A haplotype (q.v.) on the short arm of chromosome 6. Encodes the major histocompatibility complex in man and, therefore, the cell-surface molecules that present antigen to T-cells. It is highly polymorphic, making it ideal for linkage studies

In situ hybridization. This is the process of detecting target DNA or RNA in tissue sections or cell smears, by incubating with a labelled specific probe. Such probes can either be radioactively labelled (hot probe) or use cytochemical markers (cold probe). Uses include the demonstration of viral DNA within host cells

Insertion. A structural chromosomal abnormality in which material from one chromosome is inserted into a non-homologous chromosome

Intron. A segment of a gene that is initially transcribed into RNA but is then removed from the primary transcript by splicing together the exon sequences on either side of it

Inversion. A chromosomal aberration in which a segment of chromosome is inverted end-to-end

Isoalleles. 'Normal' alleles which can be distinguished from each other only by their differing phenotypic expression when in combination with a dominant mutant allele

Karyotype. The chromosome set

Kilobase. One thousand base pairs in a DNA sequence

Library. A large collection of recombinant DNA clones in which genomic or cDNA fragments have been inserted into a particular vector

Linkage. Co-inheritance of 2 or more non-allelic genes because their loci are in close proximity on the same chromosome

Linkage disequilibrium. The preferential association of a particular allele (e.g. for a disease) with a specific allele at a nearby locus more frequently than expected by chance

Locus. The position of a gene on a chromosome

Locus heterogeneity. Similar phenotypes caused by mutations at different genetic loci

Lod score. A statistical test used to show whether a set of linkage data indicates 2 loci are linked or unlinked. By convention a score of 3 (1000 : 1 odds) indicates linkage

Missense mutation. A single DNA base substitution resulting in a codon specifying a different amino acid

Mitochondrial DNA. The DNA in the circular chromosomes of the mitochondria. It is present in many copies per cell, is maternally inherited and evolves 50 to 100 times as fast as genomic DNA

Mosaic. An individual or tissue with at least 2 cell lines differing in genotype

Multiple alleles. More than 2 alleles may occur at a given locus in a population even though each normal individual can have only 2 alleles at that locus

Nonsense mutation. A single DNA base substitution resulting in a stop (termination) codon

Northern blot. A blotting technique for detecting RNA fragments by molecular hybridization
The blot reveals the size and abundance of the RNA complementary to the probe used. See also Southern blot and Western blot

Nucleosomes. The basic structural units of chromatin. Each consists of 146 b.p. of DNA wrapped around a core of 8 histone molecules

Oligonucleotide probe. Synthesized single-stranded DNA or RNA sequence to which labels can be added for use in dot-blots or in situ hybridization

Oncogenes. Genes whose aberrant activity promotes malignancy. C-onc genes are cellular genes, whereas v-onc genes are introduced from outside by a virus

p-. The designation for the short arm of a chromosome (from 'petit')

Penetrance. The frequency of expression of a genotype. A non-penetrant trait is not expressed in the phenotype

Peptide fingerprint. The chromatographic pattern of peptides obtained after partial hydrolysis of a protein or polypeptide. The technique can also be applied to DNA or RNA

Phenotype. The individual produced by the interaction between the genotype and the environment

Plasmid. Extrachromosomal circular DNA molecules often bearing antibiotic resistance genes and propagated in bacteria. They are used in recombinant DNA technology as vectors to carry cloned DNA segments

Pleiotropy. The production of multiple effects by a single gene

Point mutation. Substitution of a single base pair in a nucleic acid sequence

Polygenic. Determined by many genes at different loci, with small additive effects

Polymerase Chain Reaction (PCR). A technique used in DNA analysis which allows amplification of a particular sequence of the genome, producing multiple copies for analysis by hybridization, restriction enzyme digestion and electrophoresis. It depends on specific oligonucleotide primers (which determine the site of amplification) and repeated cycles of replication by a heat stable enzyme (taq polymerase)

Primary transcript. The direct RNA transcript of a gene, containing both introns and exons (q.v.)

Primer. A short sequence (usually 20 to 50 b.p.) complementary to one strand of DNA providing a free 3'-OH at its terminus, where DNA polymerase (e.g. taq polymerase) can act to produce a complementary strand

Proband (Propositus, index case). The family member who first presents with a given trait

Probe. A portion of single-stranded nucleic acid (DNA or RNA) labelled isotopically or non-isotopically and used to hybridize to specific nucleic acid sequences

Prokaryotic cell. A unicellular organism such as a bacterium with no nuclear membrane separating the DNA from the cytoplasm

Promoter. A sequence region which fixes the site of initiation of transcription and controls mRNA quantity

Proto-oncogenes. Normal genes which if amplified, mutated, rearranged or picked up by a retrovirus may give rise to oncogenes

Pseudogenes. DNA sequences which have undergone one or more mutations during evolution which have rendered them incapable of producing a protein product

q-. Designation for the long arm of a chromosome

Recombinant chromosome. A chromosome in an offspring that has a genotype not found in either parent

Recombinant DNA technology. Techniques whereby DNA from a gene from one organism is inserted into the genome of another organism

Recombination. The formation of new combinations of linked genes by crossing over between their loci

Renaturation. The reassociation of complementary single strands of nucleic acids into double-stranded helical forms

Restriction enzymes. Endonucleases purified from bacteria that can cut double-stranded DNA at a specific nucleotide sequence

Restriction fragment length polymorphism (RFLP). A variation in DNA sequence that alters the length of a restriction fragment produced by an endonuclease. The variations may be simple point mutations or VNTRs (q.v.). RFLPs provide convenient markers for linkage analysis

Restriction map. A map of a DNA sequence, usually in base pairs, indicating the location of restriction sites

Retrovirus. An RNA virus that encodes reverse transcriptase so that it is transcribed into DNA on entering a host cell

Reverse genetics. The application of human gene mapping to clone the gene responsible for a disease when no information about the biochemical basis of the disease is available

Reverse transcription. Synthesis of DNA on a template of RNA by reverse transcriptase

RNA. Ribonucleic acid, has 3 forms:

  (i) messenger RNA is the template for polypeptide synthesis
 (ii) transfer RNA brings activated amino acids into position along this template
(iii) ribosomal RNA is a component of ribosomes which functions as a non-specific site of polypeptide synthesis

Segregation. The separation of allelic genes at meiosis

Sex chromatin (Barr body). A chromatin mass in the nucleus which represents an inactive X chromosome. It is absent in the male

Sex-limited. A trait expressed only in one sex though the gene determining it is not X-linked

Sex-linked. A trait expressed by a gene on the X chromosome

Somatic cell gene therapy. Insertion of new DNA material into a particular tissue in such a way that the DNA does not enter the germline

Southern blot. A technique developed by Edward Southern for transferring (blotting) DNA fragments separated by gel electrophoresis to a nitrocellulose filter, on which DNA fragments can then be identified by their hybridization to radioactive probes (see also Northern and Western blots)

Taq polymerase. Heat stable DNA polymerase that enables multiple rounds of denaturation and polymerization in the PCR reaction

Transcription. Synthesis of single-stranded RNA from a double-stranded DNA template catalyzed by RNA polymerase

Transfection. Transfer of a specifically altered gene or part of a gene into a cell

Transgenic. Containing foreign DNA in the germline

Translation. The process of synthesis of protein on the mRNA template

Triplet. 3 successive bases in DNA or RNA which code for a specific amino-acid

Triploid. A cell or individual with 3 times the normal haploid chromosome number

Trisomy. The presence of 3 of a given chromosome instead of the usual pair, as in trisomy 21 (Down's)

Variable number of tandem repeats (VNTRs). These are variable length regions in DNA which can alter the length of a restriction fragment

Vector. A DNA segment capable of autonomous replication. In cloning, the vector is the plasmid, cosmid or bacteriophage used to replicate or amplify the DNA sequence of interest that is ligated into it

Western blot. A blotting technique for detecting proteins, using an immunological method

Zygote. The fertilized ovum

HISTOCOMPATIBILITY (HL-A) ANTIGENS (also called the major histocompatibility complex, MHC)

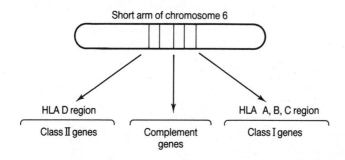

Short arm of chromosome 6

HLA D region — Class II genes

Complement genes

HLA A, B, C region — Class I genes

Histocompatibility antigens are present on all tissues of the body. There are two series of antigens determined serologically at each of 2 loci on chromosome 6, and a further series of antigens determined only in the mixed lymphocyte reaction. Some diseases occur more frequently in association with certain HL-A antigens, possibly due to related immune response (IR) genes. Foreign antigens (e.g. viral) are recognized by T lymphocytes only if certain class II MHC molecules are present on the antigen-presenting cell. The MHC can thus 'restrict' the immune response to foreign antigens

SOME HLA ASSOCIATIONS

A3, B7, B14	Haemochromatosis
B8, DR3	Autoimmune hepatitis Sjøgren's syndrome SLE Dermatitis herpetiformis Graves' disease Myasthenia gravis Addison's hypoadrenalism Idiopathic membranous glomerulonephritis
B8, DR3, DR7, DQW2	Coeliac disease
B27	Ankylosing spondylitis (> 90%) Other seronegative spondarthropathies
DR2	Narcolepsy (100%) Multiple sclerosis Goodpasture's syndrome
DR2, DR3	Primary sclerosing cholangitis
DR4	Rheumatoid arthritis
DR4, DR3	Insulin dependent diabetes mellitus

Pyrexia and hypothermia

Causes of PUO
1. Infection
   (i) Exclude:
   tonsillitis, pneumonia, pyelonephritis, cholangitis, enteric fever, septicaemia, pus under tension, endocarditis, pericarditis, etc.
   (ii) Consider possibility of:
   TB, brucellosis, parasites (worms, malaria, etc.) and viral infections (esp. HIV)
2. Collagen-vascular disease
3. Malignancy (e.g. hypernephroma, lymphoma, hepatoma or atrial myxoma)
4. 'Silent' myocardial or pulmonary infarction
5. Drug hypersensitivity prior to onset of rash
6. Rarities: familial Mediterranean fever, Whipple's disease, Fabry's, Weber–Christian, Kikuchi's, etc.
7. Psychogenic and hysteria
8. Munchausen's syndrome

HYPOTHERMIA

Causes of hypothermia
1. *Decreased heat production*
   (i) Hypothyroidism or hypopituitarism
   (ii) Hypoglycaemia or severe malnutrition
   (iii) Inactivity—crippling disease, Parkinsonism, depression, etc.
2. *Increased heat loss*
   (i) Exposure in a cold environment
   (ii) Erythroderma
   (iii) Alcoholic intoxication
   (iv) Paget's disease
3. *Failure of thermoregulation*
   (a) *Central*
       (i) 'Stroke' (especially intracranial bleed in infants)
       (ii) Drugs, e.g. barbiturates, phenothiazines
       (iii) Uraemia or diabetic ketoacidosis

(iv) Moribundity
(v) Miscellaneous neurological diseases, e.g. Wernicke's
encephalopathy, diencephalic epilepsy,
craniopharyngioma
(b) *Peripheral* (autonomic dysfunction)
Any severe illness

Complications of hypothermia
1. *Pulmonary*
Bronchopneumonia, pulmonary oedema or hypotension may
be induced by fast rewarming
2. *Cardiac*
Ventricular fibrillation or bradyarrhythmias (J waves)
3. *Metabolic*
Hypoxia, hypercapnia, acidosis, hypoglycaemia or fluid shifts
4. *Gastrointestinal*
Haemorrhagic erosions, gastric or colonic dilatation, ileus,
pancreatitis
5. *Others*
Disseminated intravascular coagulation
Microinfarcts in many tissues
Muscular rigidity

Clinical chemistry

NORMAL ADULT RANGE FOR LABORATORY ASSAYS

The International System of Units (SI units) is now established in British and European laboratories, though North American laboratories continue to use the Imperial Units, which are empirical. SI units are preferred by the Royal Colleges for examination questions. Submultiples of SI units use the following prefixes:

Factor	Name	Symbol
10^{-1}	deci	d
10^{-2}	centi	c
10^{-3}	milli	m
10^{-6}	micro	μ
10^{-9}	nano	n
10^{-12}	pico	p
10^{-15}	femto	f

Blood
Alanine amino-transferase, up to 45 Reitman–Frankel units/ml
Alkaline phosphatase, 25–85 IU/100 ml (3–13 KA units/100 ml)
Ammonia, 23–47 μmol/l (40–80 μg/100 ml)
Amylase, up to 200 Somogyi units
Aspartate amino-transferase (AST, SGOT), females 9–25 μ/l, males 10–40 μ/l
B_{12}, 100–1000 ng/l
Bilirubin (total), up to 17 μmol/l (up to 1 mg/100 ml)
Calcium, 2.2–2.7 mmol/l (9.0–10.8 mg/100 ml)
Ionized calcium, 1.1–2.4 mmol/l (4.5–5.6 mg/100 ml)
Cholesterol: desirable, less than 5.2 mmol/l; high, more than 6.2 mmol/l
Copper, 12–25 μmol/l (75–160 μg/100 ml)
Cortisol 9 am, 190–690 nmol/l (7–25 μg/100 ml)
12 midnight, 80–190 nmol/l (3–7 μg/100 ml)
Creatine kinase, M.B. fraction <7.5 μg/l, (7.5 ng/ml)
Creatinine, 53–106 μmol/l (0.6–1.2 mg/100 ml)

Electrolytes
  Na, 136–149 mmol/l (or mEq/l)
  K, 3.8–5.2 mmol/l (or mEq/l)
  Cl, 100–107 mmol/l (or mEq/l)
  Bicarb, 24–30 mmol/l (or mEq/l)
Ferritin, 20–400 µg/l
Fibrinogen, 2–4 g/l (200–400 mg/100 ml)
Folate, 6–21 µg/l
Glucose (fasting venous sample, glucose oxidase assay),
    3.0–5.3 mmol/l (55–95 mg/100 ml)
Haptoglobin, 0.7–1.3 g/l (72–125 mg/100 ml)
HGH, 1–5 µIU/ml during G.T.T.
Immunoglobulins
  IgG, 80–160 mg/l
  IgA, 14–42 mg/l
  IgM, 5–19 mg/l
  IgD, 0.03–4 mg/l
Insulin, 0–208 pmol/l (0–29 µU/ml)
Lactic dehydrogenase, 55–200 IU/l (110–400 spectrophotometric
units/ml)
Phosphate, 0.8–1.4 mmol/l (2.5–4.5 mg/100 ml)
Protein (total), 60–80 g/l (6–8 g/100 ml)
    Albumin, 33–46 g/l (3.3–4.6 g/100 ml)
Red cell folate, 160–640 µg/l
Testosterone, total (in female), 0.7–3.1 nmol/l (20–90 ng/dl)
Total T3, 1.2–3 nmol/l
Total T4, 51–154 nmol/l
TSH, 0.5–5 mU/l
TIBC, 45–72 µmol/l (250–400 µg/100 ml)
Triglycerides (fasting), 0.3–1.7 mmol/l
Urea, 2.5–6.6 mmol/l (15–40 mg/100 ml)
Uric acid, up to 0.4 mmol/l (up to 6 mg/100 ml)

Blood gases (arterial)
Oxygen 12–15 kPa (90–100 mmHg)
Carbon dioxide 4.5–6.1 kPa (34–46 mmHg)

Urine (assuming a normal diet)
Specific gravity 1.008–1.030
pH 4.8–7.5
Ascorbic acid, 114–170 µmol/24 h (20–30 mg/24 h)
Calcium, 2.5–7.5 mmol/24 h (100–300 mg/24 h)
Chloride, 100–180 mmol/24 h (or mEq/24 h)
Creatinine, 9–17 mmol/24 h (1–2 g/24 h)
5HIAA, 16–73 µmol/24 h (3–14 mg/24 h)
Phosphate, 16–48 mmol/24 h (0.5–1.5 g/24 h)
Potassium, 25–100 mmol/24 h (or mEq/24 h)
Sodium, 100–200 mmol/24 h (or mEq/24 h)

VMA, 10–40 μmol/24 h (2–8 mg/24 h)
Urea, 250–500 mmol/l (10–40 g/24 h)

CSF
Chloride, 120–128 mmol/l (or mEq/l)
Glucose, 2.5–3.9 mmol/l (45–70 mg/100 ml)
Protein, up to 0.4 g/l (up to 40 mg/100 ml)
Lymphocytes, up to 4/cu mm

SPECIAL TESTS

Glucose tolerance test
Normal limits, using 75 g oral load with venous plasma
measurements

	Fasting (mmol/l)	2 hours post-glucose (mmol/l)
Normal	<5.6	<7.8
Diabetic	>7.8	>11.1

Creatinine clearance should exceed 100 ml/min

Ammonium chloride test for urinary acidification
(using 0.1 g/kg body wt of NH_4Cl)
Urine pH should fall below 5.3 and urinary titratable acidity should
exceed 25 μEq/min

Phosphate excretion index (PEI)
The ratio $\dfrac{\text{phosphate clearance}}{\text{creatinine clearance}}$ is dependent upon the plasma

PO_4 level

The PEI indicates the extent to which this ratio departs from the
predicted normal for a given plasma PO_4 level

i.e. PEI = Observed $\dfrac{CP}{CCr}$ – 'Normal' $\dfrac{CP}{CCr}$

where the normal $\dfrac{CP}{CCr}$ = 0.055 plasma PO_4 – 0.07

On a normal diet, PEI should be 0 ± 0.09

Xylose absorption test (using 25 g xylose)
The 5 hour urinary excretion of xylose should exceed 6 g. This is a
test of upper small intestine function. It is usually normal in
pancreatic disease
Pancreolauryl test. The pancreas-specific cholesterol ester
hydrolase in pancreatic juice hydrolyses the test compound,
fluorescein dilaurate, releasing water soluble fluorescein. This is

absorbed and excreted in the urine. A control capsule containing fluorescein only is taken on the second day.

$$\frac{\text{Dye excreted from test capsules}}{\text{Dye excreted from control capsules}} \times 100 \text{ should exceed } 30\%$$

Fat absorption test on normal diet
Total faecal fat over 5 days should not exceed 5 g/day

Dexamethasone suppression test
1. Dexamethasone **0.5 mg** 6 hourly for 2 days
   Normally urinary 17-hydroxycorticoids suppress to less than 2.5 mg/24 h
   In adrenocortical hyperplasia there is less suppression
2. Dexamethasone **2.0 mg** 6 hourly for 2 days
   With bilateral hyperplasia there is suppression to less than 50% of the base-line assay
   With adenoma or carcinoma there is less suppression
Note that exceptions may occur

Short Synacthen test
Synacthen 250 μg i.m. is injected and serum cortisol is measured at 30 and 60 min. Serum cortisol should rise to over 200 nmol/l above basal level, or to a peak exceeding 600 nmol/l

Depot Synacthen (5 h)
As for the short test, except that 1 mg Synacthen is injected, with a further test at 5 h. Serum cortisol should exceed 1000 nmol/l

Depot Synacthen (72 h)
As for the 5 h test, except that the injection and tests are repeated on 3 successive days. Serum cortisol should exceed 1000 nmol/l on day 3. Rising values may indicate adrenal insufficiency

Insulin tolerance tests (Dangerous in hypopituitarism)
Standard. After an overnight fast, soluble insulin is given i.v. in a dose of 0.1 U/kg and blood glucose, cortisol and GH are measured every 30 min for 2 h. GH conc should exceed 10 μIU/ml in at least one post-insulin specimen
Augmented ITT (for acromegaly) uses 0.3 U/kg and should not be performed if hypopituitarism is suspected

TRH test
200 μg of TRH is injected as a rapid i.v. bolus and TSH is measured at 20 and 60 min. In normal people, TSH rises to between 5 and 25 mU/l with the 20 min value exceeding the 60 min value
An exaggerated response indicates hypothyroidism
An impaired response indicates hyperthyroidism or hypopituitarism

Prothrombin times

Recommended therapeutic ranges for INR:

Deep vein thrombosis prophylaxis	1.5–2.5
Deep vein thrombosis prophylaxis in hip surgery, fractured femur, etc.	2.0–3.0
Deep vein thrombosis and pulmonary embolism Prosthetic heart valves Arterial disease, e.g. myocardial infarction	2.0–4.5

Statistics

Ben Burton

Terms and tests used

Population
A specialized term applied to an aggregate of things being studied,
e.g. a particular group of patients, a number of surgical operations
or a group of blood tests

Random sample
A sample selected from a population by a random, i.e. unbiased,
process

Mean ($\bar{x}$)
The average of a set of values (i.e. sum of values divided by the
number of values)

Median
The middle value of a set of values, (i.e. the number of
observations less than the median is the same as the number of
values above it)

Normal distribution
(also called a Gaussian distribution or a normal curve):

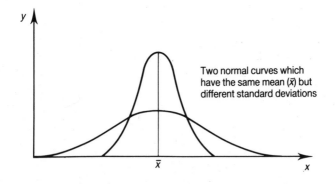

Two normal curves which
have the same mean ($\bar{x}$) but
different standard deviations

A normal curve is a continuous distribution of values which if plotted graphically would have a symmetrical bell-shaped curve, which is uniquely defined by its mean and its standard deviation (q.v.). Many biological characteristics, e.g. height, IQ, haemoglobin levels, conform fairly closely to a normal distribution

Variable
A quantity that can assume any value within a specified set of values. A variable may be *discrete* (e.g. a number of patients, which must be a whole number), or *continuous* (e.g. their heights, which are limited only by the accuracy of the method of measurement)

A *dependent* variable is one which is at least partly determined by one or more independent variables

An *independent* variable is one which establishes the value of another variable when a defined relationship exists between them

Variance
The average squared deviation of a set of values from their mean. Where each individual observation is x,
the mean is $\bar{x}$,
and the number of observations is n,
the variance is given by the equation
$[\Sigma (x - \bar{x})^2] \div (n - 1)$

Standard deviation (SD)
The square root of the variance. This gives an idea of how widely the range of values is scattered about the mean

Thus if the observed values were 22, 24, 26, 28 and 30, $\bar{x}$ is 26, and n is 5

The variance is then $[(-4)^2 + (-2)^2 + (0)^2 + (4)^2 + (2)^2] \div 4$

$= 40 \div 4 = 10$

The SD is 3.16, and the SE is 1.41

If the values were 12, 14, 26, 38, and 40, $\bar{x}$ is still 26, n is 5, but the variance is 170

The SD is then 13.04, and the SE is 5.83

In a population with a normal distribution (q.v.):

Mean $\pm$ 1 SD includes 68% of the observed values

Mean $\pm$ 2 SD includes 95% of the observed values

Mean $\pm$ 3 SD includes 99.7% of the observed values

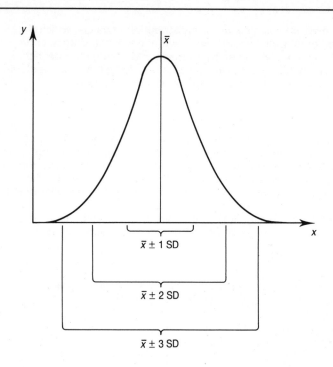

Standard error (SE)
This is the standard deviation divided by the square root of n, the number of observations. The SE of the mean of one sample is an estimate of the SD that would be obtained from the means of a large number of samples drawn from that population

P value
This is a probability limit, e.g. for a normal curve the probability that an observation will fall beyond the mean ± 2 SD is 5% or less. The P value is usually expressed as a fraction of 1 rather than as a percentage, so in this case it would be written $P < 0.05$

Confidence interval
This is the interval, as calculated from observations on a random sample, within which will lie, with a degree of probability specified in advance, the true value of a given population parameter. In other words, it gives the probability of being correct if one regards the confidence interval as containing the true value
  The *confidence limits* are defined as the boundary values of a confidence interval. Thus the mean ± 2 SD gives the 95% confidence limits for a normal distribution

Null hypothesis
The hypothesis is that there is no difference between two observed populations, and we then set confidence limits within which we regard the samples as showing no significant difference. If the difference observed is greater than these limits, the null hypothesis is unlikely to be true, and the populations are likely to be different

Correlation
The interdependence between two variables. If a change in one variable causes a change in the same direction in the second variable, the correlation is positive. If the second variable changes in the opposite direction, the correlation is negative

Correlation coefficient (r)

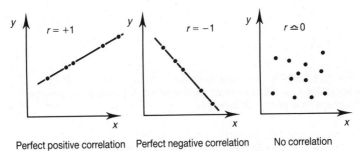

Perfect positive correlation   Perfect negative correlation   No correlation

A statistical index of the degree of linear dependence between the pair of values taken by observations of two variables. By definition, this must lie between +1 and −1, being positive if the two variables increase or decrease together, and negative if one increases while the other decreases. A zero correlation coefficient implies a complete absence of correlation

Regression equation (see Fig. on p. 246)
Correlation between two variables means that when one changes by a certain amount, the other also changes on average by a certain amount. If y is the dependent variable and x is the independent variable, the regression equation represents the change in y for any given change in x. For a straight line graph the regression equation is $y = a + bx$

t-test (Student's t-test)
A test of statistical significance which is particularly applicable to small samples (less than about 60) with a normal distribution. It involves the ratio of a sample statistic to its standard error

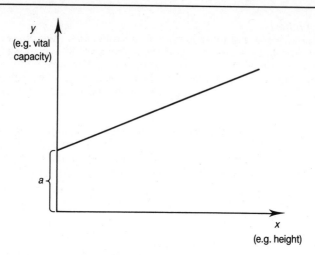

To illustrate a regression equation

Paired t test: This is used to make comparisons of paired observations, e.g. blood tests repeated before and after a certain treatment in a group of patients

Chi-square test (χ^2) (pronounced kie, as in pie)
This is used to test for differences between two independently derived proportions, e.g. to test whether the proportion of gastrectomy patients who subsequently get TB is greater than the proportion of vagotomy patients who get TB. The χ^2 test should be performed only on actual numbers of occurrences, not on percentages, proportions or means

Non-parametric tests
These are used to analyse data that do not (or might not) conform to a normal distribution. Examples include the Mann-Whitney U test and the Wilcoxon Rank Sum test

Type 1 error
An error which causes rejection of the null hypothesis when it is in fact true, e.g. it may suggest that a treatment is effective even when it is not

Type 2 error
An error which causes acceptance of the null hypothesis when it is in fact false, e.g. it may suggest that an effective treatment is not effective

Bibliography

It is unlikely that even the most assiduous of candidates will find time to study all of the following books. Special attention should be paid to the subjects in which the least clinical experience has been gained. It is more important to cover the whole of medicine superficially than to know some subjects in great detail with areas of complete ignorance in other subjects. A thorough knowledge of a small textbook will be more useful than a patchy knowledge of a large one.

For clinical examinations it is essential to read a book on the elicitation and interpretation of physical signs, e.g. *McLeod's Clinical Examination*. The British National Formulary is also strongly recommended for study.

The following Colour Atlases published by Wolfe Medical and Scientific Publications, London, provide a valuable form of vicarious clinical experience:

AIDS	C F Farthing et al
AIDS in the Tropics	M A Ansary
Bone Disease	V Parsons
Cardiology	N Conway
Cardiovascular Disease	L M Shapiro and K M Fox
Clinical Neurology	M Parsons
Dermatology	G M Levene and C D Calnan
Diabetes	A Bloom and J Ireland
Digestive System	R E Pounder
Endocrinology	D Evered, R Hall and R Greene
Eye in Systemic Disease	E E Kritzinger and B E Wright
General Medicine	M Zatouroff
Geriatric Medicine	A Kamal and J C Brocklehurst
Hand Conditions	W B Connolly
Infectious Diseases	R T D Edmond and H A K Rowland
Liver disease	S Sherlock and J Summerfield
Nutritional Disorders	D S MacLaren
Ophthalmological Diagnosis	M A Bedford
Oral Medicine	W R Tyldesley
Respiratory Diseases	D G James and P R Studdy

Rheumatology	A C Boyle
Sexually Transmitted Diseases	A Wisdom
Tropical Medicine and Parasitology	W Peters and H M Gilles
Urology	R W Lloyd-Davies et al

JOURNALS

Excellent review articles appear regularly in Medicine, Hospital Update and the British Journal of Hospital Medicine. Relevant leading articles in the British Medical Journal, The Lancet and the New England Journal of Medicine should also be read. These latter journals also contain many important original papers, and though one cannot read every paper in detail it is worth scanning each issue to pick out important advances relating to internal medicine. Every reader must develop a method which suits him or her best, but I find that the quickest way to imprint the 'message' of a paper on my memory is to read the Summary, then the Introduction (which puts the work in perspective and explains why it was done) and then reread the Summary. Examination candidates are unlikely to have time to read the Methods and Discussion of original papers, except in subjects in which they have a special interest.

Many MRCP examiners regularly read the Quarterly Journal of Medicine.

FURTHER READING

Asterisks denote larger texts and reference books.

CARDIOLOGY

*Braunwald E 1991 Heart disease: a textbook of cardiovascular medicine, 4th edn (2 vols). Saunders, Philadelphia
Julian D G, Camm A J et al 1989 Diseases of the heart. Baillière Tindall, London
Julian D G, Cowan J C 1992 Cardiology, 6th edn. Baillière Tindall, London

ELECTROCARDIOGRAPHY

Bennett D H 1989 Cardiac arrhythmias: practical notes on interpretation and treatment, 3rd edn. Butterworths, Oxford
*Goldman M J, Goldschlager N 1989 Principles of clinical electrocardiography, 13th edn. Appleton and Lange, Los Altos
Hampton J R 1992 The ECG made easy, 4th edn. Churchill Livingstone, Edinburgh
Hampton J R 1992 The ECG in practice, 2nd edn. Churchill Livingstone, Edinburgh (Hampton books are companion volumes)

CHEST DISEASE

Brewis R A L 1991 Lecture notes on respiratory disease, 4th edn. Blackwell Scientific, Oxford
*Crofton J, Douglas A et al 1989 Respiratory disease, 4th edn. Blackwell Scientific, Oxford
West J B 1989 Respiratory physiology – the essentials, 4th edn. Williams and Wilkins, Baltimore

GASTROENTEROLOGY

*Shearman D J C et al 1989 Diseases of the gastro-intestinal tract and liver, 2nd edn. Churchill Livingstone, Edinburgh
Sherlock S, Dooley J 1993 Disease of the liver and biliary system, 9th edn. Blackwell Scientific, Oxford
*Sleisinger M H, Fordtran J S 1989 Gastrointestinal disease, 4th edn (2 vols). Saunders, Philadelphia

HAEMATOLOGY

Dacie J V, Lewis S M 1990 Practical haematology, 7th edn. Churchill Livingstone, Edinburgh
Hoffbrand A V, Lewis S M 1992 Postgraduate haematology, 4th edn. Heinemann, Oxford
*Williams W J et al 1990 Hematology, 4th edn. McGraw-Hill, New York

NEUROLOGY

Morris J G L 1992 The neurology short case
*Rowland L P 1989 Meritt's textbook of neurology, 8th edn. Lea and Febiger, Philadelphia
Walton J N 1985 Brain's diseases of the nervous system, 9th edn. Oxford University Press, Oxford
Walton J N 1989 Essentials of neurology, 6th edn. Pitman, London

OPHTHALMOLOGY

Kanski J J, Thomas D 1990 The eye in systemic disease, 2nd edn. Butterworth Heinemann, Oxford

ENDOCRINOLOGY

Hall R, Besser M 1989 Fundamentals of clinical endocrinology, 4th edn. Churchill Livingstone, Edinburgh
Watkins P J 1990 Diabetes and its management, 4th edn. Blackwell Scientific, Oxford
*Wilson J D, Foster D W 1992 Williams' textbook of endocrinology, 8th edn. Saunders, Philadelphia

RENAL DISEASE

*Brenner B M, Rector F G 1991 The kidney, 4th edn (2 vols). Saunders,
   Philadelphia
Gabriel R 1988 Renal medicine, 3rd edn. Baillière Tindall, London
Sweney P et al 1989 The kidney and its disorders. Blackwell Scientific,
   Oxford
Willatts S M 1986 Lecture notes on fluid and electrolyte balance, 2nd edn.
   Blackwell Scientific, Oxford

RHEUMATOLOGY

Dieppe P A et al 1985 Rheumatological medicine. Churchill Livingstone,
   Edinburgh
Golding D N 1989 Synopsis of rheumatic diseases, 5th edn. Wright, Bristol
*Kelley W N et al 1989 Textbook of rheumatology, 3rd edn. Saunders,
   Philadelphia
*Scott J T 1986 Copeman's textbook of the rheumatic diseases, 6th edn
   (2 vols). Churchill Livingstone, Edinburgh

DERMATOLOGY

Burton J L 1990 Essentials of dermatology, 3rd edn. Churchill Livingstone,
   Edinburgh
*Champion R H, Burton J L, Ebling J 1992 Textbook of dermatology,
   5th edn (4 vols). Blackwell Scientific, Oxford

VENEREOLOGY

Adler M W 1990 A.B.C. of sexually transmitted diseases, 2nd edn. British
   Medical Association, London

TROPICAL DISEASE

*Adams A R D, Maegraith B G 1989 Clinical tropical diseases, 9th edn.
   Blackwell Scientific, Oxford
Bell D 1990 Lecture notes on tropical medicine, 3rd edn. Blackwell
   Scientific, Oxford

IMMUNOLOGY

*Male D et al 1991 Advanced immunology, 2nd edn. Gower, London
Roitt I M 1991 Essential immunology, 7th edn. Blackwell Scientific, Oxford
A Lancet Series (15 contributors) 1989 Peptide regulatory factors. Arnold,
   London

EMERGENCY MEDICINE

Haddad L M, Winchester J F 1990 Clinical management of poisoning and
   drug overdose. Saunders, Philadelphia
Salter R H 1987 Common medical emergencies. Wright, Bristol

AIDS

*Saude M A, Volberding P A 1990 The medical management of AIDS,
   2nd edn. Saunders, Philadelphia
Mitchell D M, Woodcock A A 1990 AIDS and the lung. British Medical
   Association, London
Penneys N S 1989 Skin manifestations of AIDS. Martin Dunitz, London

CLINICAL CHEMISTRY

Zilva J F, Pannall P R 1988 Clinical chemistry in diagnosis and treatment,
   5th edn. Arnold, London
Scully R E et al 1992 Normal reference laboratory values. New England
   Journal of Medicine 327: 718–724

GENETICS AND MOLECULAR BIOLOGY

Brock D 1993 Molecular genetics for the clinician. Cambridge University
   Press, Cambridge
Emery A E H, Mueller R F 1992 Elements of medical genetics, 8th edn.
   Churchill Livingstone, Edinburgh
Gelehrter T D, Collins F S 1990 Principles of medical genetics. Williams and
   Wilkins, Baltimore

STATISTICS

*Hill A B, Hill I D 1991 Bradford-Hill's principles of medical statistics. Arnold,
   London
Swinscow T D V 1983 Statistics at square one. British Medical Association,
   London

DRUGS AND DRUG REACTIONS

Davies D M 1991 Textbook of adverse drug reactions, 4th edn. Oxford
   University Press, Oxford
*Dukes M N G et al 1992 Meyler's side-effects of drugs, 12th edn. Elsevier,
   Amsterdam
Rubenstein D et al 1991 Lecture notes on drugs and therapeutics. Blackwell
   Scientific, Oxford

RADIOLOGY

Chapman S N R 1990 Aids to radiological differential diagnosis, 2nd edn. Baillière Tindall, London

GERIATRICS

Blackburn A M 1989 Geriatric medicine. Heinemann, London
Coni N et al 1988 Lecture notes in geriatrics, 3rd edn. Blackwell Scientific, Oxford

GENERAL

Hind C R K 1992 X-ray interpretation for the MRCP, 2nd edn. Churchill Livingstone, Edinburgh
Munro J, Edwards C 1990 McLeod's clinical examination, 8th edn. Churchill Livingstone, Edinburgh
Rubenstein D, Wayne D 1991 Lecture notes on clinical medicine, 4th edn. Blackwell Scientific, Oxford
Sawyer N, Gabriel R, Gabriel C 1993 300 medical data interpretation questions for the MRCP, 4th edn. Butterworth Heinemann, Oxford
Spalton D J et al 1993 100 case histories for the MRCP, 3rd edn. Churchill Livingstone, Edinburgh
*Weatherall D J, Ledingham D G G, Warrell D A 1987 Oxford textbook of medicine, 2nd edn. Oxford University Press, Oxford

Index

Abdominal pain, 48
Abscess, lung, 37
Absent jerks with
    extensor plantars, 130
Absent spleen, 74, 88
Acanthosis nigricans, 197
Acid-base balance, 176
Acidosis, 176, 177
ACTH, 137
Active chronic hepatitis, 66
ADH, 180
Adrenal hyperplasia, 151
Adrenal insufficiency, 151
Adult respiratory distress
    syndrome, 35
AIDS
  cutaneous, 213, 214
  definition, 215
  gastrointestinal, 59
  neurological, 107
  pulmonary, 36
  -related complex, 216
  rheumatic, 194
Airways
  obstruction, 27
Alcohol
  effects, 102
  flushing, 198
Aldosterone, 152, 153
Alkalosis, 177
Allergic reactions, 223
Alopecia, 205
Alpha-fetoprotein, 67
Amenorrhoea, 141
Amino-aciduria, 174
Ammonium chloride test, 239
Amnesia, 106
Anaemia, 75–79
Anatomy
  basal arteries of brain, 122

facial nerve, 118
lungs, 22
peripheral nerves, 127
Angioid streaks, 110
ANCA, 193
Angiotensin, 152
Ankylosing spondylitis, 181
Anticardiolipin antibody, 93
Anticoagulants, 99
Anticytoplasmic antibodies, 193
Antidiuretic hormone, 180
Antinuclear antibodies, 193
Antithrombin III, 92
Aortic regurgitation, 10
Aplastic anaemia, 81
ARDS, 35
Arginine vasopressin, 180
Argyll Robertson pupils, 130
Arrhythmias, 1–3
Arterial pulse, 1
Arteritis, 194
Arthritis, infective, 187
Asbestos, 32
Ascites, 57
Aseptic meningitis, 102
Aspergillus, 38
Atrial fibrillation, 2
Atrophic spleen, 74, 88
Autoimmune hepatitis, 66

Backache, lumbar, 182
Basal arteries of brain, 122
Bibliography, 247
Biliary cirrhosis, 63
Biliary obstruction, 63
Biochemical tests, 237–240
Bladder, neurological control, 127
Bleeding, 95
Blindness, 110

Blind loop syndrome, 53
Blisters, 208
Blood gases, 25, 238
Blood transfusion, 99
B lymphocytes, 219
Bone disease, 160
Bone pain, 182
Bowel ischaemia, 49
'Bowing' of tibia, 164
Bradycardia, 2
Brain death, 100
Bronchial carcinoma, 38
Bronchiectasis, 29
Bronchitis, 27, 28
Broncho-pulmonary eosinophilia, 38
Broncho-pulmonary segments, 22
Bulbar palsy, 104
Bundle branch block, 19

Calcification, abdominal, 54
Calcification, intracerebral, 108
Calcification, soft tissue, 163
Calcitonin, 159
Calcium homeostasis, 158
Calcium pyrophosphate
    arthropathy, 184
Calculi, renal, 171
Cannon waves, 3
CAPD, 167
Carcinoma bronchus, 38
Carcinoma liver, 67
Carcinoma, non-metastatic
    complications, 129, 196
Carcinomatous neuropathy, 129
Cardiac arrest, 15
Cardiac axis, 17
Cardiac catheterization, 21
Cardiomegaly, 12
Cardiomyopathy, 12
Carpal tunnel syndrome, 188
Cataract, 109
Catheterization, cardiac, 21
Cell surface markers, 218
Cerebral ischaemia, 121
Cervical sympathetic pathway, 116
Charcot joint, 130
Chest X-ray, 41
Cheyne-Stokes respiration, 26
Chi-square test, 246
Cholecalciferol, 158
Cholestasis, 63
Chondrocalcinosis, 184

Chorea, 132
Cigarette smoking, 30
Cirrhosis, 62
'Click-murmur' syndrome, 10
Clubbing, 39
CNS disseminated lesions, 108
Coagulation, 94–98
Coma, 101
Complement, 221
Compliance, 25
Confidence interval, 244
Constipation, 58
Continuous ambulatory peritoneal
    dialysis, 167
Continuous murmurs, 7
Cord compression, 125
Cor pulmonale, 30
Correlation, 245
Cough, persistent, 30
Crackles, 26
Cranial nerves, 112
Crohn's disease, 55
Cryoglobulinaemia, 190
Cyclo-oxygenase pathway, 223
Cytokines, 218

Dark urine, 174
Deafness, 120
Death, 100
Deficiency
    B$_{12}$, 53, 79
    D, 158
    folate, 79
Dementia, 105
Dermatomes, 124
Dexamethasone suppression test,
    240
Diabetes insipidus, 139
Diabetes mellitus
    causes, 145
    complications, 145
    definition, 144
    and pregnancy, 147
Dialysis, 165
Diaphragm, 125
Diarrhoea, 50
Diastolic murmurs, 7
Diffusion, 24
Disseminated CNS lesions, 108
Disseminated intravascular
    coagulation, 97
Dissociated anaesthesia, 126

Dropped beats, 2
Drug-induced
  eye disease, 111
  haemolysis, 76–78
  hypertension, 17
  liver disease, 68
  pulmonary disease, 33
  renal disease, 175
  skin disease, 209
Dwarfism, 144
Dysarthria, 104
Dysphagia, 44
Dysphasia, 104
Dysphonia, 105
Dystrophy, sympathetic, 188

Ectopic humoral syndromes, 157
Eczema, 209
Effusion, pleural, 34
Ejection sounds, 5
Electrocardiography, 17–20
Emphysema, 27, 28
Encephalopathy, hepatic, 64
Endocrine neoplasia, 156
Endogenous opiates, 137
Eosinophilia, 38, 83
Epilepsy, 107
Extensor plantars, 130
Eye movements, 118

Facial nerve, 118
Facial pain, 119
Factor VIII, 95
Familial jaundice, 69
Fanconi syndrome, 173
FEV, 23
Fibrillation, 2
Fibrinogen deficiency, 97
Fibrosis, pulmonary, 32
'Flitting' arthritis, 186
Flushing, 198
Folate deficiency, 79
Frontal 'bossing', 163

Galactorrhoea, 140
Gastrectomy complications, 48
Gastric cancer, 47
Gastric secretion, 45, 46
'Gay bowel' syndrome, 59
Gene probes, 228

Genetic terms, 225
Geniculate herpes, 119
Giddiness, 121
Gingival swelling, 44
G6P dehydrogenase def., 78
Glasgow coma scale, 101
Glomerulonephritis, 168
Glucose tolerance test, 239
Glycosylated haemoglobin, 146
Gonorrhoea, 216
Gout, 181, 185
Gut flora, 53
Gut hormones, 51
Gynaecomastia, 140

Haematemesis, 47
Haemochromatosis, 68
Haemodialysis, 165, 166
Haemoglobinuria, 174
Haemolytic anaemia, 76–78
Haemophilia, 95
Hand muscle wasting, 128
Headache, 108
Heart
  block, 3
  failure, 11
  murmurs, 6–8
  muscle disease, 13
  sounds, 5
Heinz bodies, 75
Hemianopia, 114
Hepatitis, 66
Hepatic cancer, 67
Hepatic encephalopathy, 64
Hepatic osteodystrophy, 161
Hepatocyte injury, 65
Hepatomegaly, 60
Hermaphrodites, 143
Hirsutism, 204
Histocompatibility antigens, 233
HLA antigens, 233
Hodgkin's disease, 84
Horner's syndrome, 116
Hot joint, single, 186
Howell-Jolly bodies, 75
Hydrocephalus, 109
Hyperaldosteronism, 153
Hypercalcaemia
  causes, 161
  ECG changes, 20
  tests, 162
Hypercalciuria, 162

Hyperdynamic circulation, 1
Hypergammaglobulinaemia, 219
Hypergastrinaemia, 46
Hyperkalaemia, ECG changes, 19
Hyperlipoproteinaemia, 149, 150
Hypermobile joints, 187
Hypernatraemia, 178
Hyperparathyroidism, 162
Hyperpigmentation, 202
Hypersplenism, 88
Hypertension
  portal, 64
  pulmonary, 16
  systemic, 17
Hyperthyroidism, 155
Hypertrichosis, 205
Hypertrophic cardiomyopathy, 12
Hypertrophic osteoarthropathy,
  39
Hypertrophy, ventricular, 18
Hyperuricaemia, 185
Hyperventilation, 26
Hypoadrenalism, 151
Hypoalbuminaemia, 56
Hypocalcaemia
  causes, 161
  ECG changes, 20
Hypochlorhydria, 47
Hypochromic anaemia, 75
Hypogammaglobulinaemia, 219
Hypoglycaemia, 147
Hypogonadism, 142
Hypokalaemia, 19
Hypokalaemic acidosis, 178
Hypomagnesaemia, 179
Hypomelanosis, 203
Hyponatraemia, 178
Hypophosphataemia, 162
Hypopituitarism, 138
Hypoprothrombinaemia, 98
Hyposplenism, 88
Hypothalamic hormones, 136
Hypothermia, 235
Hypothyroidism, 154
Hypoventilation, 25
Hypoxaemia, 25

Iliac fossa mass, 54
Immunoglobulins, 219
Immune deficiency, 219
Inappropriate ADH secretion, 180
Inclusion bodies, 75

Industrial chest disease, 31
Industrial skin disease, 212
Infarction
  cerebral, 122
  intestinal, 49
  myocardial, 14, 18
Infective arthritis, 187
Innocent murmurs, 8
Insulin-like growth factors, 138
Insulin tolerance test, 240
Interleukin, 218
Intersexual states, 143
Interstitial nephritis, 170
Intracranial pressure, 116
Intravascular coagulation, 97
Iritis, 110
Irregular pulse, 2
Ischaemia
  bowel, 49
  cerebral, 121
  myocardial, 14, 18

Jaundice
  drug induced, 68
  familial non-haemolytic, 69
  with uraemia, 62
JVP, 4, 5
Juxtaglomerular apparatus, 153

Kidneys
  cystic, 173
  large, 172
  small, 172
Kobner phenomenon, 212
Korsakoff psychosis, 104

Lactic acidosis, 177
Leg ulcers, 207
Leukaemias, 85
Leukaemoid reaction, 82
Leukocytosis, 82
Leuko-erythroblastic anaemia, 82
Leukopenia, 80
Lipoproteins, 148
Lipoxygenase pathway, 224
Liver failure, 61
Liver transplant, 71
Liver tumours, 67
Lumbar backache, 182

Lung
 abscess, 37
 anatomy, 22
 volumes, 23
Lupus erythematosus, 192
Lymphadenopathy, 42, 83, 216
Lymphocyte deficiency, 219, 220
Lymphocytosis, 82
Lymphokines, 218

Macrocytic anaemia, 79, 80
Malabsorption, 51
Malignancy
 bronchial, 38
 gastric, 47
 liver, 67
 melanoma, 212
 oesophageal, 45
 skin changes, 196
Marrow depression, 80
Marrow infiltration, 80
Mass in R iliac fossa, 54
Mediastinal masses, 40
Megaloblastic anaemia, 79
Meningitis, aseptic, 102
Metabolic bone disease, 161
Methaemoglobinaemia, 75
MHC molecules, 233
Microangiopathic haemolytic
  anaemia, 78
Mitral incompetence, 9, 10
Mitral stenosis, 9
Mitral valve prolapse, 10
Monocytosis, 83
Mononeuritis multiplex, 129
Multiple endocrine adenomatosis,
  156
Murmurs, 6–8
Muscular dystrophy, 133
Mydriasis, 117
Myeloproliferative disease, 85
Myocardial infarction
 complications, 14
 ECG changes, 18
Myopathy, 133
Myotomes, 124
Myotonia, 133

Nails, 206
Necrotizing vasculitis, 194
Nephrocalcinosis, 171, 172

Nephrotic syndrome, 169
Neuroleptic drugs, 131
Neurological complications of:
 carcinoma, 129
 diabetes mellitus, 145
Neurological terms, 134
Neuromuscular transmission, 132
Neuropathy, 127, 128, 129
Neutropenia, 80
'Normal' chest X-ray, 41
Normal distribution, 242
Normal values
 biochemical, 237
 haematological, 72
Null hypothesis, 245
Nystagmus, 119

Obstructive pulmonary disease, 27
Oculomotor palsy, 116
Oedema, pulmonary, 35
Opening snap, 5
Opiates, endogenous, 137
Opportunistic infections, 36, 59
Optic atrophy, 114
Optic neuritis, 115
Oral contraceptives, 142
Osteoarthrosis, 181, 184
Osteoarthropathy, hypertrophic, 39
Osteodystrophy, 161
Osteomalacia, 160, 182
Osteonecrosis, 187
Osteoporosis, 160, 182

Paget's disease, 182
Pain, abdominal, 48
Palmar erythema, 211
Pancreatitis, 70
Pancreolauryl test, 239
Pancytopenia, 81
Papillary necrosis, 169
Papillitis, 116
Papilloedema, 115
Papules, pigmented, 212
Paraplegia, 126
Parenteral nutrition, 56
Parkinsonism, 131
Parotid enlargement, 44
Peak flow, 23
Peptic ulcer, 48
Peptides, intestinal, 51
Pericarditis, 16

Periosteal reaction, 182
Peripheral nerves, 127
Peritoneal dialysis, 167
Persistent generalized
         lymphadenopathy, 216
Phagocyte dysfunction, 220
Phakomatoses, 196
Phosphate excretion index, 239
Photosensitivity, 201
Pigmentation, 202
Pigmented papules, 212
Pituitary hormones, 137
PiZZ, 29
Platelet defects, 91
Platelets, 89
Pleural effusion, 34
Pneumoconiosis, 31
Pneumonia, slow resolution, 36, 37
Pneumothorax, 33
Polycystic kidneys, 173
Polycythaemia, 86, 167
Polydipsia, 179
Polyendocrine deficiency, 156
Polymerase chain reaction, 231
Polyuria, 179
Porphyria, 199–201
Portal hypertension, 64
Post. inf. cerebellar thrombosis, 123
Posterior pituitary, 139
Precocious puberty, 143
Proptosis, 155
Prostaglandins, 223
Protein-losing enteropathy, 57
Prothrombin, 98, 241
Proximal myopathy, 134
Pruritus, 211
Pseudobulbar palsy, 104
Pseudogout, 184
Psoriatic arthritis, 184
Ptosis, 116
Puberty, 143
Pulmonary
   abscess, 37
   compliance, 25
   diffusion, 24
   embolism, 20
   fibrosis, 32
   hypertension, 16
   oedema, 35
Pulse, 1
P value, 244
Pyrexia of unknown origin, 235
Pyuria, 170

QT, long, 4, 20

Radiology
   chest, 41
   joints, 181
   kidneys, 172
   skull, 163
Ramsay-Hunt syndrome, 119
Raynaud's phenomenon, 189
Red cell inclusion bodies, 75
Red cell shape, 73
Reflexes, 123, 130
Regression test, 245
Renal
   calculi, 171
   failure, 165
   osteodystrophy, 161
   toxins, 175, 176
   tubular disorders, 173
   vein thrombosis, 169
Renin, 152, 154
Residual volume, 24
'Respirator lung', 35
Respiratory distress syndrome, 35
Retinal haemorrhage, 110
Retrobulbar neuritis, 116
Rheumatic fever, 8
Rheumatoid disease, 181, 190
Rheumatoid factor, 192
Rinne's test, 120

Schilling test, 53
Scotoma, 114
Scleroderma, 198
'Shock', 15
'Shock lung', 35
Short stature, 144
Shoulder-hand syndrome, 188
Sick sinus syndrome, 2
Sideroblastic anaemia, 76
Sinoatrial disorder, 3
SI units, 237
Sjøgren's syndrome, 192
Skin changes in malignancy, 196
Skin test, 223
Skull X-ray, 163
Sodium retention, 179
Soft-tissue calcification, 163
Speech defects, 104
Spinal cord, 123

Spirometry, 23
Splenectomy, 88
Splenomegaly, 87
Splenic atrophy, 74, 88
Spondyloarthritis, 183
Squints, 117
Stagnant bowel, 53
Standard deviation, 243
Statistics, 242
Stiffness, 188
Stomatitis, 43
Stones, renal, 171
Student's t test, 245
Sudek's atrophy, 188
Superficial reflexes, 123
Supraventricular tachycardia, 20
Sympathetic pathway, 116
Synacthen test, 240
Syncope, 14
Syphilis, 217
Systemic hypertension, 17
Systemic lupus, 192
Systolic murmurs, 6

Tachycardia, 1, 20
TBG, 156
Tendon reflexes, 123, 130
Thalassaemia, 78
Thoracic outlet syndromes, 189
Thrill, 7
Thrombocytopenia, 89
Thrombocytosis, 91
Thrombosis, 92
Thyroid-binding globulin, 156
Thyroid function tests, 154–156
Tibial 'bowing', 164
T lymphocytes, 219
Transfusion, 99
Transient ischaemic attacks, 121
Translucencies in skull X-ray, 163
Transport defects, 173
Tremor, 130
Triple rhythm, 6
t-test, 245
T$_3$ toxicosis, 155
Tubular disorders, renal, 173
Tumours

bronchial, 38
gut endocrine, 51
liver, 67
Tunnel vision, 113
T waves, 19

Ulcerative colitis, 54
Ulcers, leg, 207
Upper zone shadowing, 42
Urine, dark, 174
Urinalysis, 238
Uveitis, 110

Vagotomy, 48
Valsalva manoeuvre, 11
Valve closure, 5
Valvular disease, 11
Vasculitis, 194
Venous pulse, 4, 5
Venous thrombosis, 92
Ventricular failure, 12
Ventricular filling sounds, 6
Ventricular pre-excitation, 3
Vertigo, 121
Vessel defects, 93
Visual field defects, 112
Vital capacity, 23
Vitamin deficiency
B$_{12}$, 53, 79
D, 158
Vitamin D synthesis, 158
Vitiligo, 203
Vomiting, 46
von Willebrand's disease, 95

Wasting of hand muscles, 128
Weber's test, 120
Wheezes, 26
Willis, circle of, 122
WPW syndrome, 3
WR, 217

Xanthomas, 150
Xylose absorption, 239